your

best

skin

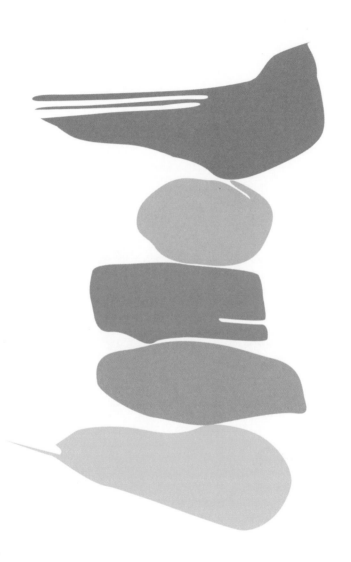

your

the science of skincare

best

skin

Hannah English

Hardie Grant

BOOKS

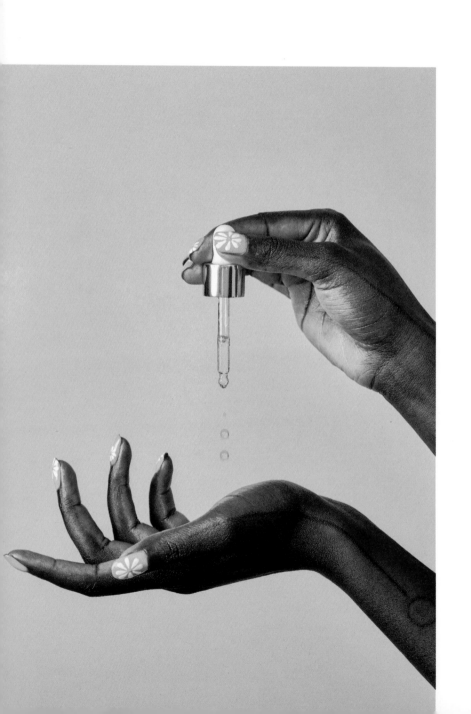

Contents

Introduction

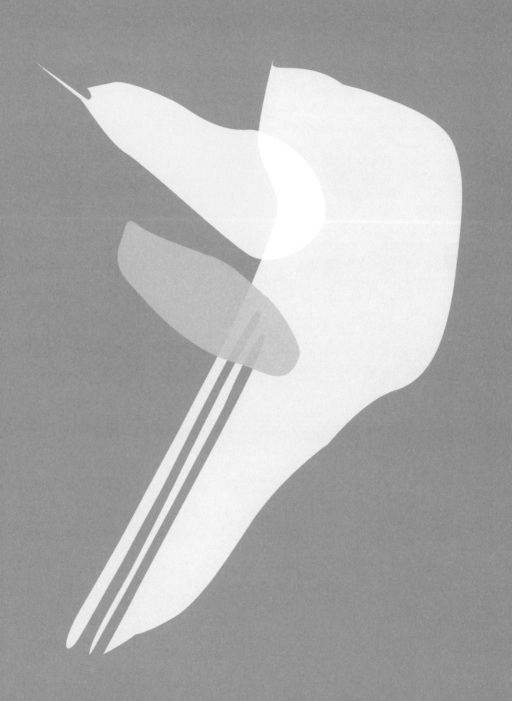

01

Hannah's story

[CHAPTER 1]

Like more than 90%[1] of teenagers, I had acne throughout late primary and high school. I tried to punish my skin into shape with harsh and stripping products, used a foaming acne cleanser, and was too scared to moisturise in case I broke out. I couldn't understand why my acne wouldn't clear up. I thought that thorough cleansing would clear the acne because my skin must be dirty. Sound familiar?

My acne did clear up when I was 19, but it came back in my mid-20s. Sigh. Contrary to popular belief, a lot of people do not 'grow out of it'. Adult acne affects 64% of people aged 20–29 and 43% aged 30–39.[2]

If I had a party on the weekend, I'd attack spots using a scrub or a squeezing tool. Of course, this made it worse. I put toothpaste on spots after reading about it in a magazine, and one time I even used Borax – a house and laundry cleaning product. It's used for cleaning so maybe it would 'clean' my skin? Unfortunately not. It gave me a chemical burn, and it *definitely* made the spot worse.

At the time, my parents insisted all would be OK and that the acne was due to changing hormones. It was, but it was still painful and I had terrible self-esteem. This is not uncommon – skin conditions are linked to issues with mental health[4] and body image,[5] and there is even an emerging field in medicine called psychodermatology,[6] combining a doctor's experience in dermatology with an understanding of mental health.

Breaking out does not mean your skin is dirty, nor does it mean that *you* are dirty. It's a medical condition, much like a headache, and it can be managed. I'd love never to see the word 'dirt' in marketing copy for a face wash again. What dirt? Did you dive into a garden bed?

Although my skin has never truly been oily, I moved on to a 3-step skincare system designed for oily skin. But almost any skin type can break out, not just oily skin. Naturally, using a harsh skincare system twice daily and once again neglecting to moisturise did me no favours, and left my skin angry and stripped of its natural defences.

Classmates commented on my breakouts in a less-than-kind way and I had a couple of partners (whose opinions I gave more time to than I should have) who would criticise my skin, teeth and weight. That's a discussion for another day but if your partner treats you this way: Dump! Them! Immediately! Do not pass GO, do not collect $200, just block their number. All of this led to bouts of low self-esteem in my teens to early 20s, as you'd expect.

The '00s were a different time, which ... is something people always say before they try to justify something awful that used to be ingrained. It was trendy to be sample size, breakouts were not seen in media or advertising, and tabloid journalism consisted of unflattering swimsuit photos of women along with comments about their cellulite (which is completely normal by the way) – the perfect recipe for body dysmorphia, distorted self-image and eating disorders.

I came to deeply dislike the use of 'before and after' photos for weight loss, procedures, skincare and makeup. While they can be used scientifically if photographed in the exact same conditions or using a special camera, in advertising the two images are often so clearly different. The 'after' photo is shot in a studio with makeup and great lighting – and almost definitely retouched in post-production. You can't compare yourself to that.

Even though body acceptance has come a long way, these attitudes are still prevalent today in beauty and fitness. We've moved from diet culture to wellness culture, but it's the same thing in a different outfit – 'you need to lose weight' is now packaged as 'everything must be clean, pure and natural'. Both are rubbish. You are valid at any weight, and striving towards wellness leaves behind those who can't, such as those with a chronic illness. You are valid, 'well' or 'unwell'. This moving target intentionally makes us feel bad about ourselves and our lives, to encourage us to buy more *stuff*.

But ... I've always loved beauty. I started wearing makeup at an early age – 10 years old – and wanted to be a makeup artist even though people insisted, 'You're too smart for beauty'. This is in itself a problem. There are many smart, hardworking scientists, businesspeople and beauty therapists involved in the BIG business of beauty.

One Christmas, my aunt gifted me a copy of *Don't Go to the Cosmetic Counter Without Me* by Paula Begoun. It changed my life. Paula's book got me excited about the science behind beauty and the development of skincare, and showed me that you can use your understanding of science and your skin to decide whether or not a product will work for *you*. In my years of trying and reviewing products, I can tell you that some people will love and get fabulous results from products that I *hated* on my own skin.

I'd always enjoyed and had a natural aptitude (or what we now know as ADHD hyperfocus) for science class, so it was a no-brainer to put my two favourite things together. After a couple of tries at university (studying media and then fashion styling), I decided to study science, intent on understanding the research behind beauty and what makes the ingredients do what they do. I chose Pharmaceutical Science because pharmacology is the study of our bodies and how different substances affect them, right down to the molecular level. Any substance that alters the function of a bodily process works like a drug, so it makes sense to learn about medical science and pharmacology to address the health of your skin. My university studies taught me how to examine scientific journal articles, and working in pharmaceutical trials helped me to understand the work that goes into collecting good-quality evidence.

These days, I use my science background and industry experience to try out products and assess skincare claims, to help cut through all of the buzzwords and more-more-more marketing, so we can all find our best skin. I consult on communications and product development for beauty brands, helping them choose ingredients and testing finished formulas on myself. I also review products for social media and publications, trying and comparing them and communicating how they interact with the skin (not just my own) in-depth.

Now, in my early 30s, my skincare has taken a turn towards 'anti-ageing' … but this terminology doesn't sit well with me. I know we're all afraid of showing our mortality, but I also know that looking like myself only a few years older is hardly the worst thing in the world. Throughout this book, I'll do my best to be specific and say exactly what I mean. I'll address the causes of fine lines or hyperpigmentation rather than use the blanket term 'ageing'. I've also seen the phrases 'authentic ageing' and 'well-ageing', but I don't love those either. There is no obligation to age well, or authentically. You can age as inauthentically as you like. Because who is the judge of that? What's the benchmark? Let's just keep our skin happy and functional and enjoy ourselves and our lives.

Let's not assign a moral value like 'good' or 'bad' to our skin as we tend to internalise this kind of messaging and think of *ourselves* as 'good' or 'bad' as a result. Then we punish our skin when it really needs some love. If you have acne or another skin condition, your skin isn't *bad*, it's just not functioning as well as it could be. I'd rather build towards being happy and healthy and that's exactly what we're going to do together.

So, think of me as your informed older sister. I harbour no judgement − only acceptance. I've made the mistakes so you don't have to. I'm here to talk to you and share everything I know …

Because a lot of us don't have access to a doctor, dermatologist, beauty therapist or dermal clinician.

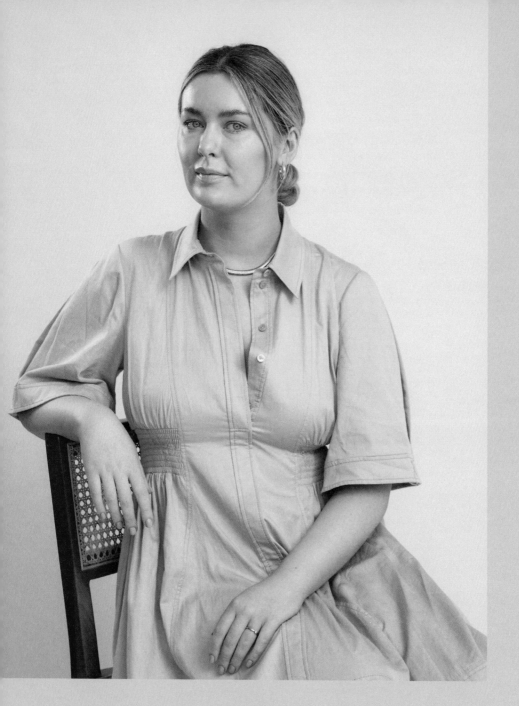

HANNAH'S STORY

Because I don't want you to be spoken to by people in your life the way I was, and I don't want you to speak to yourself the way I did.

Because I want you to be armed with the facts next time you go to your favourite beauty retailer, to decipher the advertising speak, make informed purchasing decisions and not waste your time or money. Ever again.

Because I want you to understand your skin … and yourself.

Now on to your head start, courtesy of yours truly.

Your skin

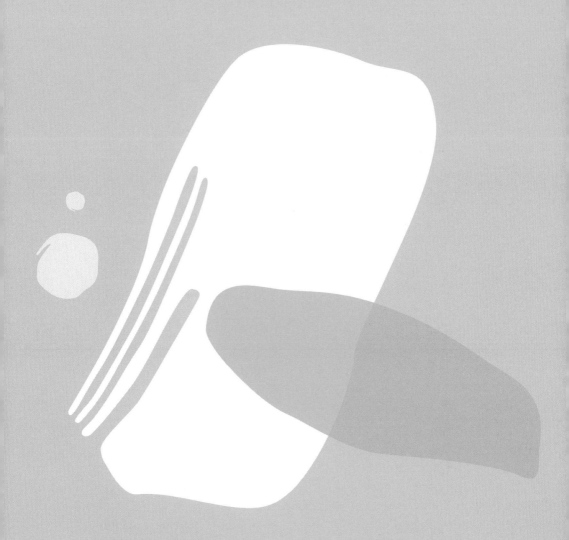

What is skin anyway?

[CHAPTER 2]

Skin is the largest organ in the body, so it makes sense for us to care for it in the same way we would care for our heart through exercise. It's important that we chat about the biology and biological function of skin, because it takes all of the stress and judgement out of the equation. Your cells and body are just doing what they do and you can help them along, if you want, with skincare.

This chapter has a few diagrams and gets a little sciencey, but don't worry, I'm not your mean high school science teacher in chino shorts and knee socks. I firmly believe a lot of the issues that people have with science come from the way it's delivered. We'll take it slow and there'll be no walls of text here. You can do it – I promise.

Your skin's job

Your skin is literally the barrier between the inside of your body and the outside environment, and a key component of your immune system. Simply put, it keeps your bones, organs and the water you need in, and the germs and sun out, and it keeps you warm and cool. Skin also generates vitamin D (more on that in Chapter 5), and it even receives and communicates signals for temperature, pain, pressure, touch, and the presence of chemicals and change in pH. These signals travel to your brain via nerves.

Understanding your skin's function as a barrier is the key to supporting and looking after it. It acts as a barrier from UV, germs, water and other environmental challenges. It also protects against foreign substances – even medicines must be designed specially to penetrate skin. It's not easy.

Face vs body

Skin on the face is different to the skin on the body. It's thinner (specifically in the dermis), and there are more sweat and oil glands. Your face, neck, scalp and chest have between 400 and 900 oil glands per square centimetre, while other parts of the body have 100 or less oil glands per square centimetre (and none on the palms of your hands and soles of your feet).[7]

Skin is thinner and drier in your eye area and it's more sensitive. It tends to be the first place that skin changes as we age thanks to our constant squinting, blinking and facial expressions. Skin around the jawline, neck and upper lip is more sensitive to hormones, which is why we grow hair there and why these areas can be prone to acne. The skin on the lips is thin and doesn't moisturise itself, but it has more nerve endings so it's more sensitive to touch. It's important to protect your lips from the sun.

Skin on the palms of the hands and soles of the feet has an extra layer of epidermis called the stratum lucidum, which makes it thicker. There's no hair on the palms and soles, and thus no oil glands. There are, however, lots of nerve endings, giving us a more precise sense of touch.

We also have different types of sweat glands and different types of sweat. Eccrine sweat is secreted all over the body and is mostly water and electrolytes. This type of sweat cools us down.

After puberty, we start to make apocrine sweat, which is secreted from the underarm and groin areas. This is emotional sweat and it contains lipids, steroids and proteins. This is the kind of sweat that mostly contributes to body odour.

Let's talk about structure

There are three layers to your skin: the epidermis at the top (on the outside), the dermis in the middle and the hypodermis underneath. There are also different types of cells and other substances present in the skin.

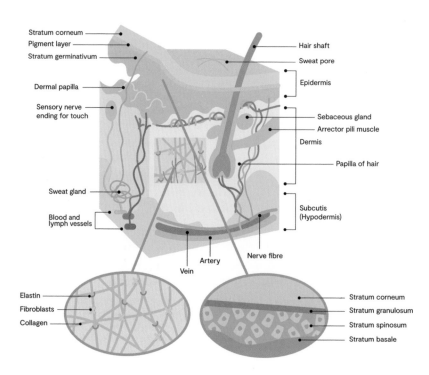

WHAT IS SKIN ANYWAY?

Epidermis

The epidermis is the top layer of your skin and it's there to keep water in and the environment out. There are four layers within the epidermis (see opposite) (but five layers on the palms and soles) and several cell types are found here. Let's meet the relevant ones.

Keratinocytes make up 90% of the cells in the epidermis and they produce proteins called keratin (also found in hair and nails) and filaggrin. Their life cycle is 24–40 days.[8] That's how long it takes for a skin cell to 'turn over', to generate in the basal layer, fill with keratin and migrate to the top layer, releasing barrier lipids (waxy fats that help to keep water in and bad bacteria out) as they go. At the top layer, keratinocytes are fully cornified/flattened/full of keratin and are called 'corneocytes'. This transformation and shedding process will take longer as things start to slow down in your body over time, but it can be helped along with skincare.

Corneocytes are keratinocytes at the end of their life cycle. There are 15–20 layers of corneocytes in the stratum corneum, surrounded by your skin's barrier lipids. Think of it as a brick wall: the corneocytes are the bricks and the lipids are the mortar. Together, they make up the skin's barrier. The corneocytes are nearly ready to shed and come off naturally in a process called desquamation (or when you exfoliate). When they come off, this signals the lower layers to make more keratinocytes.

Melanocytes exist in the basal layer (stratum basale) of the epidermis, with the new keratinocytes. They make the pigments for your skin and hair and transfer brown spots (melanin) to surrounding keratinocytes. They live for at least 3–5 years.[9] These are our target when treating hyperpigmentation.

The following figure shows the top layers of the epidermis acting as your skin's barrier. If the barrier is disrupted (from harsh cleansing, for example), it's easier for water to escape and irritants to get in.

Other substances in or on the epidermis include the microbiome, barrier lipids, sweat, sebum, the skincare you've applied and the air pollution stuck to your skin.

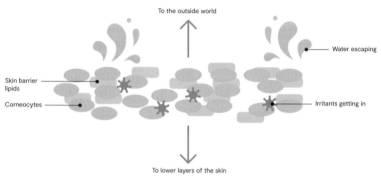

To the outside world

Water escaping

Skin barrier lipids

Corneocytes

Irritants getting in

To lower layers of the skin

The **microbiome** refers to the microorganisms (or microbes) living on and in our skin. It's a blend of bacteria, fungi (like yeasts) and viruses, found mostly in the epidermis and hair follicles. There are around 1000 species of bacteria on human skin.[10] The bacteria are mostly helpful or harmless and help to fight off the bad bacteria by eating the nutrients and starving them, influencing the immune system or producing molecules to harm them.

The bacteria on your armpit will differ from the bacteria on your face because they like different conditions. This variation in bacteria is why our underarms and feet have a different odour. As for acne bacteria, they're on everyone's skin but only sometimes cause problems (for the lucky ones).

The microbiome is influenced by many things – pollution, skincare, medication, pH, the body's immune system ... the list goes on. It also influences things in turn, including our immune system and conditions such as eczema, acne, rosacea and psoriasis. The skin microbiome is an emerging area of research.

Dermis

The dermis is the layer below the epidermis and is much thicker. It is a structural, functional layer of connective tissue, meaning it connects things together. This is where collagen is made, so if a product is designed to 'stimulate collagen' or 'firm skin', the active ingredients need to penetrate the dermis. Your skin's blood vessels sit in this layer, along with nerve endings, sweat glands, oil glands and hair follicles (pores). The dermis is mostly made up of proteins and other cell types.

Fibroblasts make your skin's collagen, elastin, and cushioning water-grabbing molecules such as hyaluronic acid.

Macrophages are part of your immune system and engulf and digest foreign things. If they can't digest something, they can fire off free radicals and contribute to inflammation.

Mast cells are also part of the immune system and are involved in allergic reactions. The granules contain histamine, which is released when an allergen is detected. Histamine creates symptoms associated with allergic reactions such as swelling, heat, itching and hives.

Other substances found in the dermis include collagen and elastin (woven together), which are proteins, and a cushiony gel made up of hyaluronic acid, water and salts.

Collagen is like a strong rope or fibre that your skin (specifically fibroblasts) weaves together to make it thick and strong. Collagen is also found in other parts of the body, such as the bones, eyes, cartilage and gums.

Elastin is another protein that is very elastic. It's what makes your skin bounce back when you move it. It's interwoven with collagen to make it flexible and lives a long time in your body – a lifetime, in fact. (We make new elastin but still keep a lot of the old elastin.)

Elastin is also found in your blood vessels and bladder, because those need to be flexible too.

Hyaluronic acid is a special molecule that varies in size. It's a chain of sugars that attracts water to form a cushiony gel. If you put just 1 g of hyaluronic acid into 100 mL of water, it will become a gel — it can hold so much water. Your body breaks down and makes new hyaluronic acid every day, to help repair wounds, plump up skin, and cushion in between cells and other structures.

Hypodermis

The hypodermis lies under the dermis and it stores fat to cushion your bones and organs, and keep you warm. Fibroblasts and macrophages are found in this layer along with adipocytes, the fat-storing cells.

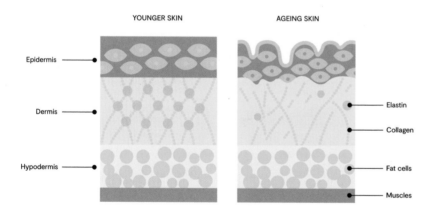

WHAT IS SKIN ANYWAY?

pH

Your skin's pH should be between 4.8 and 5.7. Therefore, knowing the pH of skincare is important for a few reasons:

— Products with a very low pH will result in a chemical burn.
— Products with a very high pH are caustic, such as drain cleaner and bleach.
— Bad bacteria like a higher pH.
— Water is a pH of 7 (neutral), so a cleanser should have a pH of 7 or lower.

Ideally, your skincare products will have a pH below 7, but not lower than 3.5 — with the exception of acid exfoliants. Anything higher than pH 7 and your barrier is at risk. Anything lower than 3.5 and, you guessed it, your barrier is at risk — not to mention the potential irritation. (We'll chat more about this in Chapter 6.)

In the pH scale on the following page, you can see that soap has a high pH of 10, which is why it's not recommended to cleanse with soap. Detergent also has a high pH of 11, which is why detergent makes your hands feel dry. Products that fall outside the ideal skin pH range of 4.8–5.7 (such as a chemical peel (pH 2–3) and hair removal cream (pH 12) should be used strictly according to instructions.

pH Scale

ACIDIC **0** ● Battery Acid

1 ●

Stomach Acid (1.5-3)

2 ● Lemon Juice

● Chemical Peel (2-3)

3

● Orange Juice

4

5 ● Black Coffee

● Skin (4.8-5.5)

6 ● Urine

● Milk (6.5) / Saliva (6.7)

NEUTRAL **7** ● Water

● Blood (7.4)

8 ● Sea Water

9 ● Baking Soda

10

● Soap (10-12)

11 ● Detergent

12 ● Hair removal cream, perming solution

13 ● Bleach, oven cleaner

ALKALINE **14** ● Drain cleaner

Key takeaways

— Your skin is a barrier that keeps your organs in and the environment out.

— If the barrier is disrupted, it's easier for water to escape and irritants to get in.

— There are different cells in the skin that do different things, and your skincare has to reach them to treat them.

— Like the rest of your body, the skin is a delicate ecosystem that must be respected.

Skin types

[CHAPTER 3]

The skin is a living, breathing organ. Just like any other organ. And, as such, it changes. All the time. Is your skin oilier in the summer, but drier in winter? Your skin's behaviour and condition changes multiple times every day and over your lifetime. It's common for your skin to become more dull, sensitive and dry as you age. And you can have normal or dry skin and still break out. So what even *is* your skin type?

Skin type categories are reductive. They were designed to categorise people and sell products, and they miss a lot of important information. We love nuance in this house, and to really know your skin and what is best for it, you need to go deeper than your existing assumptions about your skin type. Assuming that all people with a shiny T-zone have oily skin will only get you into trouble. Maybe your skin is a little oily but also dehydrated and craving water?

Categorising by skin type can be helpful to a certain extent and an easy way to communicate (at a high level) what's going on with your skin. Use it as a starting point, but always ask more questions.

—

Most people have combination skin, with multiple concerns in different places.

In this chapter, we'll talk through some common skin concerns, which will be followed by a comprehensive skin quiz. I encourage you to understand the skin concerns and think about which may apply to you.

Fitzpatrick scale

The Fitzpatrick scale was developed in 1975 to catalogue how skin reacts to phototherapy, and is one medical way to classify your skin's colour and reaction to the sun based on the amount of melanin in your skin. Some skin conditions are more common in dark skin tones (e.g. post-inflammatory hyperpigmentation), medium skin tones (e.g. melasma) and light skin tones (e.g. rosacea).

Like many other facets of society, dermatology has a problematic history of systemic racism,[11] and the Fitzpatrick scale initially didn't include the darker skin types 5 and 6. Historically, skincare research was only conducted on Fitzpatrick skin types 1–4 (i.e. white to medium/olive skin tones). Advertising also hasn't traditionally catered to medium to dark skin tones, which still continues to this day. When treating skin, it is imperative to know how to accurately, safely and effectively treat skin of all colours.

FITZPATRICK SKIN TYPES[12]		
Skin type	**Typical features**	**Tanning ability**
I	Pale white skin, blue/green eyes, blond/red hair	Always burns, does not tan
II	Fair skin, blue eyes	Burns easily, tans poorly
III	Darker white skin	Tans after initial burn
IV	Light brown skin	Burns minimally, tans easily
V	Brown skin	Rarely burns, tans easily
VI	Dark brown or black skin	Never burns, always tans

Skin concerns

Sensitive skin

Globally, the prevalence of self-reported 'sensitive' skin is estimated at 50% or more.[13] However, the use of the word 'sensitive' isn't medical and instead acts as a catch-all term for skin conditions such as irritant contact dermatitis (a reaction that's not related to allergy), allergic contact dermatitis (e.g. allergies to bandages or grass), hives, rosacea, eczema, genetically dry skin and naturally thinner skin.

You might think you have sensitive skin if your skin is reactive to products or sensations. To make your skin more comfortable, incorporate gentle skincare products into your routine to strengthen your barrier.

Oily vs dry skin

The oiliness of your skin is influenced by genetics, age, climate, sex hormones (specifically androgens) and the wrong skincare products. Conversely, truly dry skin is characterised by a lack of oil, which can leave it cracked or flaky as it struggles to retain water and reinforce the barrier.

A lot of people mistake their skin type for oily if they're prone to breakouts, but acne can happen to those with dry skin as well. Breakouts are about the thickness of the oil as well as the amount of oil. Treating your whole face as if it's oily when it's actually normal to dry can worsen the breakouts and prevent your skin from getting what it needs.

Dehydrated skin

While dry skin needs oil, dehydrated skin needs water (or you might be extra lucky and need both). As we get older, skin becomes drier regardless of our sun exposure. How well you retain water and stay naturally moisturised is an indicator of your skin's barrier function – that is, how well it is keeping the water in. If your skin feels tight or flaky but still oily, it needs water as well as help hanging on to that water.

Hyperpigmentation

If your skin is great at making melanin (pigment), then it's similarly great at making excess pigment when stressed – from the sun, a breakout, friction, a rash – leaving you with dark spots. Accumulative sun exposure results in dark spots, which usually become visible from your late 20s.

How well do you know your skin?

It's now time to take the skin quiz to get a better understanding of your skin concerns. Each section of the quiz is designed to get you thinking about your own skin and how it behaves. There's no right or wrong. There's no boxing anyone into oversimplifying their skin.

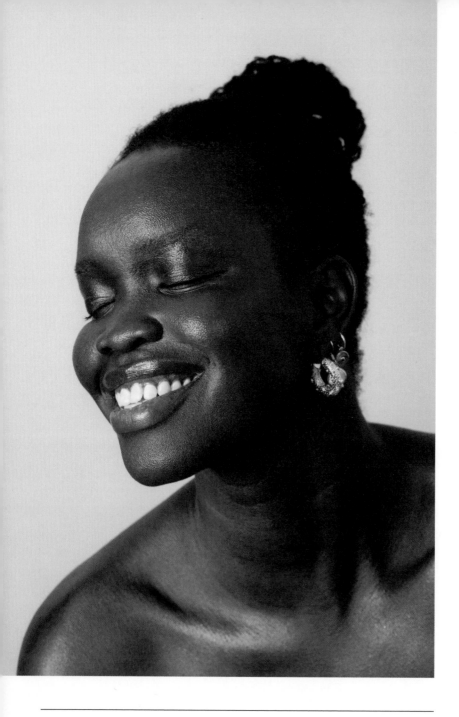

SKIN TYPES

QUIZ: HOW WELL DO YOU KNOW YOUR SKIN?

Oily/dry/dehydrated

1. What happens an hour after you wash your face and don't moisturise?
a) It becomes oily very quickly
b) It feels comfortable but not shiny
c) It feels tight*
d) It is rough and flaky

2. Does your skin look shiny in photos?
a) Always
b) Sometimes
c) Never

3. Are your pores visible?
a) All over
b) Only on nose, chin and forehead, but not the cheeks
c) No

4. What does your skin feel like at the end of the day?
a) Oily all over
b) Oily forehead, nose, chin; normal cheeks
c) Normal forehead, nose, chin; dry cheeks
d) Smooth and hydrated
e) Dry and thirsty all over

5. If you wear makeup, what happens by the middle of the day?
a) Makeup is shiny
b) Makeup is shiny and separated*
c) Makeup is smooth
d) Makeup is cracked, creased and flaky

6. Do you have clogged pores?
a) Yes, all over
b) T-zone only
c) No

Answers
1. a) oily b) average c) average/dehydrated d) dry
2. a) oily b) average/combination c) dry
3. a) likely oily or aged/lost elasticity b) combination c) average to dry
4. a) oily/dehydrated b) combination c) combination, but more dry d) average e) dry/dehydrated/both
5. a) average to oily b) dehydrated but oily c) average d) dry/dehydrated/both
6. a) most people do b) combination skin c) likely dry skin or blessed by genetics

* These answers are indicators of dehydration.

Sensitivity

1. **Do skincare products irritate your skin or cause it to break out?**
   a) Often
   b) Sometimes
   c) Rarely
   d) Never

2. **Do you have rosacea? Does anyone in your family?**
   a) Yes, I do
   b) Yes, in my family
   c) Maybe
   d) No

3. **Do you have eczema or another skin condition? Does anyone in your family?**
   a) Yes
   b) Maybe
   c) Family
   d) No

4. **Do perfumed products make your skin break out, or feel dry or itchy?**
   a) Often
   b) Sometimes
   c) Rarely
   d) Never

5. **Does your face or neck go red after exercise, or when angry, embarrassed or stressed?**
   a) Often
   b) Sometimes
   c) Never

6. **Do you get flushed after consuming any particular food and drink (e.g. spicy food, alcohol)?**
   a) Often
   b) Sometimes
   c) Rarely
   d) Never

Answers
1. a) barrier is compromised, skin is very sensitive and/or using the wrong products b) barrier is compromised and/or using the wrong products c) likely happens when barrier is compromised d) yay!
2. a) do not use too many products or harsh products b) be careful and use SPF c) go see your doctor d) lucky you!
3. a) likely to have reactive skin so be careful with exfoliating; focus skincare on restoring and hydration b) keep an eye out; be careful with exfoliating c) may be prone in future so be gentle with skin d) lucky you!
4. a) likely to have sensitive skin b) likely to have sensitive or sensitised skin c) pretty common d) lucky you!
5. a) indicator that skin is thin or extra sensitive to stimuli b) indicator that skin is temporarily thinned or extra sensitive to stimuli c) skin is not extra sensitive to stimuli
6. a) skin is extra sensitive to stimuli b) skin may be extra sensitive to stimuli c) probably not sensitive to stimuli d) not sensitive to stimuli

Pigmentation

1. **After a pimple, cut or ingrown hair, do you get brown or purple/red spots in its place?**
   a) Brown
   b) Red/purple
   c) Both

2. **Have you developed dark spots or patches from pregnancy, hormone replacement therapy (HRT) or hormonal contraceptives?**
   a) Yes
   b) No

3. **Do you have freckles? How many?**
   a) None
   b) 1–5
   c) 5–15
   d) 16+

4. **When exposed to sun, your skin:**
   a) burns
   b) burns then tans
   c) tans
   d) tans easily
   e) never burns

5. **Do your parents have freckles or sunspots?**
   a) Yes
   b) No

Answers
1. a) prone to post-inflammatory hyperpigmentation b) prone to post-inflammatory erythema c) prone to post-inflammatory hyperpigmentation and post-inflammatory erythema
2. a) possible melasma
3. This is a scale of how prone your skin is to pigmentation.
4. This is a scale of how sun-resistant your skin is.
5. This is an indicator of whether you will develop freckles or sunspots later in life.

Over to you

Now that you understand your skin's behaviour a little better, let's talk about your skin concerns. What do you want to target with skincare? Do you want to reduce breakouts (see Chapter 11), sensitivity (see Chapter 4) or hyperpigmentation (see Chapter 13)? All of the above? Perhaps you just want to protect your skin and keep things running smoothly.

I'm often asked for 'a good moisturiser for oily skin', and it's just not that simple. Is your skin tight but still oily? Is it prone to clogged pores? Do you prefer a nourishing feeling in your moisturiser or something lighter? Are you oily all over, or just in the T-zone? Really think about what you're trying to achieve and build a skincare routine that will target your specific skin concerns.

Key takeaways

— Skin types are reductive and were
  invented to sell products.

— Most people have combination skin.

— Truly dry skin is different from
  dehydrated skin. Dry skin needs oil,
  while dehydrated skin needs water.

— Your skin is not constant and changes
  all the time. Take the quizzes in this
  chapter from time to time to see
  how your skin is behaving at that
  particular moment.

— Choose products for your skin
  concerns, *not* your skin type.

Sensitive or sensitised?

[CHAPTER 4]

Many people classify their skin as *sensitive*, yet there is no clear-cut medical definition for what that means.

I like to think of it as skin that's less tolerant and naturally more responsive or reactive to external stimuli, such as temperature, pH, skincare products, mechanical sensations such as touch (or, shock-horror, scrubbing), and even alcohol or spicy foods. It's skin with a delicate temperament.

Sensitive skin is different to skin that might be *sensitised* if it's feeling particularly reactive. For me, the biggest indicator that something is wrong is when a product that's normally fine for me to use starts to tingle, burn or sting. This means the barrier (we'll get to that in a minute) has been weakened and things are penetrating that normally wouldn't, so the nerves in your skin are firing off like alarm bells! You might notice rashes, excessive dryness, peeling, or skin feeling tight, hot or itchy. Not all skin turns red when inflamed but that can also be a sign.

What causes skin to become sensitised?

Things that can sensitise your skin or contribute to an impaired barrier include:

— sun exposure, even if you're not sunburnt
— drying cleansers and soaps
— harsh or frequent scrubbing, friction
— cleansing brushes and scratchy washcloths
— over-exfoliating with AHAs and/or BHAs, enzymes or scrubs
— overuse of active ingredients (e.g. vitamin C, vitamin A or derivatives, hydroquinone, kojic acid)
— overly astringent toners
— showers or baths that are too hot
— dry climates and low-humidity environments (e.g. air conditioning and heating).

This doesn't mean all of these things are bad for you, but they are something to be mindful of.

How to treat sensitive or sensitised skin

Here are my best tips and actions for you to take when your skin just won't behave:

— **Be militant with your sunscreen use.** This is not negotiable.
— **Cut out anything that might contribute to stress.** No actives – so no scrubs, acids, enzyme exfoliants, exfoliating cleansers or retinoids. If you find vitamin C a bit spicy, give that a rest too.

— **Use the most gentle cleanser you can.** In general, this is a great strategy for keeping your skin happy and healthy.
— **Limit variables.** Keep your skincare as simple as possible.
— **Be consistent.** Use hydrating and repairing products day and night.
— **Consider an occlusive.** An occlusive is a thick balm or ointment that forms a physical barrier, acting in place of the natural barrier. It can be incredibly healing and you only need a pea-size amount for the entire face.

ROUTINE: SENSITIVE/SENSITISED SKIN

AM

1. Gentle cleanser (optional)
2. Repair serum (optional)
3. Moisturiser
4. SPF

PM

1. Oil cleanser (optional)
2. Gentle cleanser
3. Repair serum (optional)
4. Gentle moisturiser
5. Occlusive (optional)

Continue for at least four weeks, or for as long as you need to.

Supporting and repairing your skin's barrier

Your skin's purpose as an organ is to act as a physical barrier between you and the outside world. When I refer to the barrier, I am talking about the very top layer of your skin's epidermis – the stratum corneum. The barrier keeps water in and it keeps infectious agents and environmental stressors out.

Water is essential to life and if you zoom in to your skin specifically, it's essential for all of the millions of chemical reactions happening to keep things running smoothly – making collagen, signalling to old cells that it's time to shed, preventing stress … I could go on all day.

One of the most important things to learn about your skin is how to tell when it's not doing well and how to repair it. Here's a visual of what's going on when you have a damaged barrier.

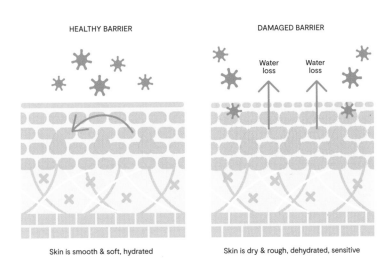

HEALTHY BARRIER

DAMAGED BARRIER

Water loss   Water loss

Skin is smooth & soft, hydrated

Skin is dry & rough, dehydrated, sensitive

See how the cells and lipids are disorganised when the barrier is damaged, letting water out and environmental stress in?

Inflammation is a cascade, with multiple cell types and chemical messengers involved, giving feedback to each other. The sooner you stop it in its tracks, the better.

Skincare ingredients that help support the barrier

Look for a few of these ingredients in your moisturiser or serum to help calm, hydrate and support the barrier.

INGREDIENT	WHAT DOES IT DO?
Ceramides	These naturally make up about 40% of your skin's barrier lipids so replenishing them with products helps strengthen your barrier.
Cholesterol	Another key component of your skin's barrier lipids, at around 25%. A strong barrier means resilient skin.
Free fatty acids	Yet another key component of your barrier lipids, at 10–15%. Specifically, you might see stearic acid, linoleic acid (an omega-6), linolenic acid (an omega-3) or palmitic acid.
Safflower oil, sunflower seed oil	Both are known to help with barrier function, with minimal allergenicity.
Phospholipids	Your body chops these up to make ceramides, which strengthen skin and help it to stay hydrated.
NMF (natural moisturising factor)	Water-grabbing molecules that help to hydrate. A product might say 'NMF' on the label, or you can look for ingredients like amino acids – specifically alanine, histidine, glutamine, serine, arginine and valine.
Electrolytes	In the same way that drinking Hydralyte rehydrates you (and replaces lost electrolytes from sweat), electrolytes will attract water and hydrate your skin.
Niacinamide	Aka vitamin B3. Has been shown to strengthen the barrier. It's also calming, reduces redness and the sensation of heat, helps with minimising the look of pores and delivers bonus anti-dark spot action.

INGREDIENT	WHAT DOES IT DO?
Panthenol	Aka vitamin B5. It helps support skin to make free fatty acids (like the ones in the barrier) and also reduces redness (and heat), stinging, burning and itching.
Hyaluronic acid	Naturally present in the dermis of your skin, it can bind to a lot of water at a time and help retain it in your skin.
Allantoin	Helps to hydrate, smooth and soothe skin. It is found naturally in comfrey root, sycamore and horse chestnut.
Beta glucan	Hydrating, soothing and protective. It is found naturally in oats and barley.
Oat	Also labelled as Avena sativa. Soothing and great for very dry and eczema-prone skin types. It also has antioxidant properties as it contains caffeic and ferulic acids.
Centella	Soothing and encourages skin to hydrate itself. It's also great for healing, with antioxidant properties.
Cucumber	Hydrating and anti-inflammatory.
Green tea	Calming to skin and can make your sunscreen work harder with its potent antioxidant activity. Look for Camellia sinensis leaf extract on the ingredient list.
Squalane	A very stable, lightweight oily liquid that helps prevent water loss and gives your skin a smoothing, moisturised effect.

MY FAVOURITE PRODUCTS
TO SUPPORT AND REPAIR SKIN

Cleansers

— Avène Extremely Gentle Cleanser Lotion
— Bioderma Sensibio H2O Micellar Water

Moisturisers

— La Clinica Deep Hydration Moisture Cream
— Beauty Bay Thirst Trap Rich Moisturiser with Oatmeal and Oat Lipid
— KraveBeauty Oat So Simple Water Cream
— Avène Skin Recovery Cream
— Bioderma Sensibio Light Moisturiser
— Bioderma Cicabio Soothing Repairing Cream

Serums

— KraveBeauty Great Barrier Relief Serum
— Apothaka Barrier Support Serum
— tbh. Skincare Rebound Serum
— Medik8 Hydr8 B5 Intense Serum
— La Clinica Hydrating and Healing Serum

Face oil and occlusives/balms

— Sunday Riley Juno Antioxidant + Superfood Face Oil
— La Roche-Posay Cicaplast Baume B5 Balm
— QV Intensive With Ceramides Sting-Free Ointment

Rosacea

Rosacea is often mistaken for acne, but using acne products to treat rosacea can make it worse. While acne symptoms and lesions are related to clogged pores, rosacea is related to an impaired barrier and damaged blood vessels – pores are not involved. Rosacea is a medical condition and can be quickly resolved with a visit to a GP or dermatologist.

Symptoms to look for include:

— flushing, stinging, burning
— inflammatory lesions that look like pimples, central to the face
— increased skin sensitivity
— visible blood vessels
— red or itchy eyes.

Here are some things you can do in the meantime to help treat rosacea:

— **Make sunscreen your best friend to prevent further damage to the barrier and blood vessels.** Collagen, elastin and hyaluronic acid help line and cushion those blood vessels, while UV and environmental stress will damage them.
— **Work on strengthening and repairing your barrier with a very simple, restoring skincare routine.** Include ingredients such as niacinamide, hyaluronic acid, ceramides and omegas in your skincare.
— **Talk to your doctor.** They can prescribe medicines and in-clinic treatments that will help keep symptoms at bay, such as anti-inflammatory and antibiotic creams, azelaic acid and vascular lasers. Lasers target the problem blood vessels, shrinking them and preventing their inflammation. Visit www.faceuptorosacea.com to help you prepare for your doctor's appointment.

One of the most important things to learn about your skin is how to tell when it's not doing well and how to repair it.

SENSITIVE OR SENSITISED?

Key takeaways

— *Sensitive* skin is skin that is less tolerant and naturally more responsive or reactive to external stimuli.

— *Sensitised* skin is skin that is temporarily feeling particularly reactive, such as when a product that's normally fine to use starts to tingle, burn or sting.

— Happy barrier, happy skin.

— There's a lot you can do to nourish your skin and work on sensitivity. Incorporate key ingredients in your moisturiser or serum to help calm, hydrate and support the barrier.

Your skincare routine

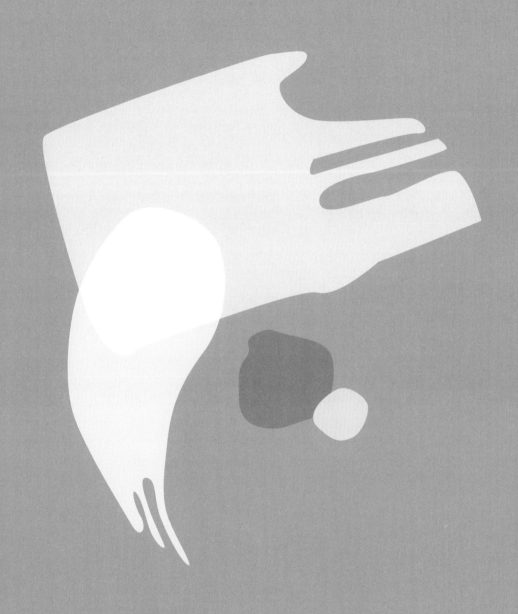

03

Sunscreen

[CHAPTER 5]

We're going to start your skincare routine right here. Because sunscreen is the single most important step. Two in three Australians are expected to be diagnosed with a form of skin cancer by age 70,[14] while one in five Americans will develop a skin cancer in their lifetime, and numbers are on the rise in the UK. There have been multiple skin cancers in my family.

If that hasn't convinced you, here are a few more reasons why you should wear sunscreen every day.

— **Sunscreen is the only true anti-ageing skincare product.** Sure, other products can help to reverse damage, but sunscreen is the only thing that actually prevents it.
— **Our skin's appearance changes drastically over the course of our lives.** This is due to a lot of things slowing down or progressively not working as well as they used to. So if I told you that 80% of these changes are thanks (but no thanks) to UV radiation and they could be managed with regular sunscreen use, you'd be keen, right? Investing in your future? Future-proofing your skin? Thought so.

- **Wearing sunscreen daily reduces your risk of skin cancer.** This is especially true in Fitzpatrick skin types 1–4, but types 5 and 6 should still wear it. If you're prone to hyperpigmentation, reducing UV exposure with sunscreen is the best treatment strategy.
- **There's nothing healthy about a tan.** Skin tanning is evidence that the sun is up to no good and sunscreen will help to minimise the damage. In skin that doesn't tan, the damage is still happening, even from the tiny amount of UV coming through your sunscreen.
- **Sun damage is cumulative.** Walking to and from the car, sitting in the car (yep, some UV can pass through windows), dashing outside to get the mail or hanging out the washing – it all adds up. In fact, if you were to have a skin cancer, the DNA mutation patterns can indicate whether it came from being badly burnt a few times, or from the day-to-day cumulative effect of sun damage. Both types of exposure can do it. So it stands to reason that both can prematurely contribute to changes in our skin, and not in a good way.
- **UV radiation is ultraviolet energy from the sun.** UV radiation is present whether or not the sun is out. I've been sunburnt on a cloudy day and had a visible tan line on my back (from my bikini top) on my skin for 3 years afterwards. It was horrific. So when I say to wear sunscreen every day, I mean: Every. Single. Day. The temperature isn't an indication of UV radiation, nor is cloud cover – there's still radiation reaching our skin and damaging it. Things like snow, sand, concrete and water all reflect UV.
- **UV radiation contributes to inflammation.** When you protect your skin from UV radiation, you're also protecting it from inflammation, and this will improve the symptoms of almost any skin condition. Hyperpigmentation? Related to heat and inflammation. Acne? Inflammation plays a key role.

Rosacea? Yep, inflammation. And damage to the structure of blood vessels is related to (you guessed it) UV exposure. Whatever your skin is doing, wearing sunscreen will help.

What is the sun up to?

The sun produces a lot of energy and UV isn't the only kind. About 50% of radiation from the sun is infrared, 40% is visible light and 10% is UV radiation. Infrared is largely felt as heat, visible light is what helps us see, and UV radiation can be further broken down into UVA, UVB and UVC.

We're going to start at the smallest, molecular level and work our way through to visible effects on the skin.

UVB

UVB is more destructive than UVA and for the most part only penetrates as far as the epidermis. This varies between light skin (more gets through) and dark skin (less gets through).[16]

When UVB hits the inside of your cells, the DNA can warp. Your body has in-built DNA repair mechanisms that can reverse the change or clip out a section of the DNA before it replicates. The problem is, these mechanisms take a lot of resources and can be overwhelmed – that's when you get sunburnt. Over time the mutations add up.

UVA

There's twenty times more UVA than UVB in sunlight,[17] and unlike UVB, UVA can penetrate through glass, such as your car or office window. UVA also penetrates past the epidermis and into the dermis, where it affects dermal fibroblasts – the cells responsible for making collagen and elastin. Again, more UVA gets past the epidermis in light skin compared to dark skin.[18]

People who used sunscreen daily showed significantly less signs of photo-ageing compared to people who used sunscreen only when they felt like it.[15]

UVA is lower energy than UVB, but it generates free radicals and thus oxidative stress. Free radicals create about 50% of UV damage to skin, with direct radiation covering the rest.[19] Their effects destabilise proteins as well as DNA, which is an issue for skin as DNA repair mechanisms are proteins. Free radicals can also damage your cells' membranes and cause DNA strand breaks.

What does this all mean? UVA and UVB work together to make a bad time for your skin.

Let's now zoom out to the cellular and structural level.

UV radiation

UV radiation inhibits procollagen production, meaning your cells aren't making as many building blocks for collagen. It directly activates inflammation, which isn't ideal, especially if your skin is already inflamed. Inflammation is exponential so the sooner you stop it, the better. UV radiation also interferes with your immune system working properly, both locally (making it harder for your body to detect skin cancers) and systemically.[20]

In sun-damaged skin, there are less blood vessels and they're not distributed evenly. That's because the UV has degraded the surrounding support structures and there's no scaffold holding them in place.[21] Yikes. How will your skin get its nutrients now?

Blue light (high-energy visible light)

Screens don't emit nearly enough blue light to cause any problems, but the sun does. We know that blue light contributes to wrinkles, loss of elasticity and hyperpigmentation (especially in Fitzpatrick skin types 3–6). Although we don't yet know *how*, we do know how to protect ourselves from its effects – by using a sunscreen formula containing iron oxides or antioxidants.[22] Iron oxides have visible yellow, red or black pigments, so they might not look as nice as a clear sunscreen.

Infrared

Infrared energy produces heat, which is partly why the sun feels warm. This is not ideal if you have melasma, a hyperpigmentation condition that's worsened by heat. With infrared, it's all about the dose and the conditions. We use near-infrared LED 830 nm in-clinic (or in an at-home LED mask) to promote healing and improve collagen quality. However, when you experience infrared alongside UV radiation, it contributes to generation of free radicals, which means your skin can't take as much UV before burning. There's good news, though – once again, you can use a sunscreen with added antioxidants to stay protected.

What does this mean for your skin?

Think about the difference in the appearance and structure of your skin in sun-exposed areas, such as the hands, compared to somewhere that sees less sun, such as the stomach.

The medical term is 'photo-ageing' and it's the most common and visible sign of accumulated UV exposure. You might see fine lines and deeper wrinkling, loss of elasticity, changes to texture and more visible pores (pore visibility is related to skin elasticity, among other things). There might also be hyperpigmentation (solar lentigines aka sunspots), damage to blood vessels which can look like all-over redness, or visible red capillaries at the surface of the skin called telangiectasias (you might know them as broken capillaries, but that's not what they are). All of these changes are largely permanent but they can be reversed a little over time with commitment to skincare and procedures. That being said, sunscreen and sun-smart behaviour are *much* easier and cheaper, I promise.

Let's talk sun protection

Researchers in the US conducted a study,[23] where participants spent 3.5 hours at the beach during the hottest part of the day. Half of the participants used only a beach umbrella and the other half used only SPF 100 sunscreen. Which group do you think got more sunburnt?

It was the beach umbrella group. Are you surprised? It's important to note that there was some sunburn in both groups, so combining sun protection methods is ideal. Wear protective clothing, sunglasses (make sure they're UV category 2 or higher)[24] and a hat. Stay in the shade and wear sunscreen (I don't wear sunscreen under clothing unless it's sheer) and try to stay out of the sun between 11 am and 3 pm because that's when UVB radiation is highest.

A note on Vitamin D

Vitamin D helps our bodies to absorb minerals such as calcium, which is part of our bones. A lack of vitamin D will have implications for the health of our bones.

Most of our vitamin D is made in our skin and it needs UVB to do this.[25] Sunscreen use will not result in vitamin D deficiency[26] (believe me, I am obsessed with sunscreen and my vitamin D levels are great). This might be because a little UV always gets through sunscreen (the same reason you can tan with sunscreen on), or it might be from not reapplying; whatever the case, unsafe sun behaviour to increase vitamin D levels is not recommended by doctors.[27] Thankfully, vitamin D is also found in food and deficiency can be addressed through diet or supplements. If you think you might be vitamin D deficient, talk to your doctor.

Sunscreen FAQs

What is sunscreen?

Sunscreen is a product applied to skin that absorbs some of the sun's radiation so your skin doesn't have to. The ingredients that do this are called UV filters. Sunscreen has been proven to reduce the risk of skin cancers and reverse sun-related skin changes.[28]

Do I need one that's natural?

No sunscreen is natural. In order to pass the regulatory testing to be sold as a sunscreen, a formula must be reproducible and manufactured in a TGA-approved facility (i.e. a lab).

What does 'SPF' mean?

SPF stands for 'sun protection factor' and is determined in a lab. Skin is exposed to a UVB lamp and the amount of UVB energy it takes the skin to burn is recorded. This is called the MED (minimal erythemal dose) – the dose of UVB your skin can take before burning. This varies between different skin tones (see Chapter 3), so as a Fitzpatrick type 2 my MED might be lower than my mum's (a Fitzpatrick type 3), but it's probably higher than my dad's (a Fitzpatrick type 1).

When sunscreens are tested to find the SPF, researchers take the amount of UV it takes to burn with sunscreen on and divide it by the amount it takes to burn without. So skin wearing an SPF of 50+ can take at least fifty times the UV.

You might have seen it explained this way: if you usually burn in five minutes, multiply that by the SPF factor of your sunscreen. So, if you have an SPF 50+, multiply five minutes by 50 and you have 250 minutes before burning.

That's kind of correct, but five minutes in June is very different to five minutes in January. And most people don't apply enough sunscreen, nor do they reapply every two hours or after swimming. Oftentimes, people get sunburn due to incorrect sunscreen use – they don't apply enough, they don't reapply or they stay in the sun past their maximum UV dose.

Lamps used in labs give off the same amount of UVB energy every time. The sun, however, is not consistent. So don't think about sunscreen as the number of minutes you can spend in the sun – that will vary throughout the day and throughout the year. Rather, practise sun-smart behaviour. Wear sunscreen (and lots of it), reapply, cover up with clothing and a hat, protect your eyes with sunglasses and stay in the shade.

—

In Australia, SPF 50+ means the sunscreen is actually SPF 60 or higher, whereas SPF 50 means it's 50–59. Lots of pressure for one little plus sign.

What about UVA?

Look for 'broad spectrum' on the sunscreen label – this means there's some UVA protection. In Australia, a sunscreen of SPF 30 or above must be labelled broad spectrum and it must have a UVA protection factor (UVAPF) of at least ⅓ of the UVB. So an SPF 30 will have a UVAPF of at least 10. I know – 10 isn't much, which is why I prefer my SPF as high as possible.

The test for UVAPF is often done by applying sunscreen to a plastic slide and measuring how much UVA passes through.

In other countries, you might see a UVAPF rating, PPD rating or PA rating to address UVA protection. In the UK, some sunscreens have a Boots UVA star rating on the packaging. The percentages are the UVA to UVB protection ratio. If a sunscreen is SPF 50 with a 5-star UVA rating, that means the UVA protection is 90–100% of 50, so between 45 and 50. Isn't it helpful!

A PPD (persistent pigment darkening) rating is like the SPF test, only subjects are measured for the UVA dose it takes to tan. For example, a PPD of 10 means that the sunscreen will multiply the UVA dose it takes you to tan by 10.

How much sunscreen is enough?

When SPF testing is carried out, sunscreen is applied at a density of 2 mg/cm² of skin, so that's how much you'll need to apply to get the labelled level of protection. If you apply less, you'll get less SPF.

But don't worry, the maths has been done for you. You need to apply 1 teaspoon (or 5 mL) for each limb, 1 teaspoon each for the front and back of your torso, and 1 teaspoon for your head and neck if you have no hair. For your face and neck, you'll need a ½ teaspoon or (2.5 mL). Your face alone is a ¼ teaspoon or (1.25 mL), but these amounts can be adjusted accordingly. (Some people measure their face with graph paper and a sheet mask to get an exact measurement.)

My moisturiser/makeup has SPF – is that enough protection?

Maybe, but it depends on how much is applied. I might have applied my skincare and makeup liberally when I was 15, but for most people, using this much of their fancy foundation or moisturiser is too expensive in the long term (and not great if you're after a more natural look). Even though my moisturiser and foundation always had SPF, my skin still became sun damaged because I hadn't applied enough.

So how much moisturiser or foundation should you apply? The recommendation is a ½ teaspoon for the face and neck (same as the recommendation for sunscreen).

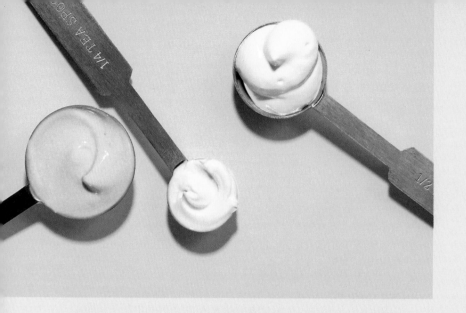

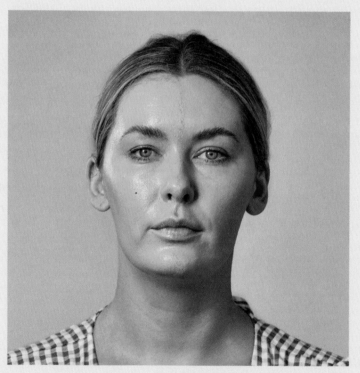

SUNSCREEN

Why do I need to reapply sunscreen?

Think about the way your makeup changes throughout the day. It's designed to form a film on your skin for even coverage but your natural oils and sweat start to break it down. The same breakdown happens to sunscreen and while it's not as immediately visible, you can end up with patchy coverage, which is why it's important to reapply sunscreen. You should reapply sunscreen every 2 hours, but studies have shown that even one reapplication throughout the day makes a difference to skin compared to only one application. And use common sense – if you're in the sun for a long time, reapply every 2 hours; if you're indoors, twice a day is plenty.

How do I reapply sunscreen if I'm wearing makeup?

It's not as difficult as it sounds. Some brands make sunscreen mists that you can use to top up your sunscreen, such as Kate Somerville (US), Labiotte (Korea), Bioderma (UK) and Naked Sundays (AU). Just be sure to use a lot as most of it ends up in the air.

And please don't use SPF powders! How can you get a ¼ teaspoon of SPF powder on your face? I reject the idea that it's better than nothing, because a false sense of security is never a good thing.

My favourite method for reapplying sunscreen over makeup is to use a liquid sunscreen, like La Roche-Posay's Anthelios Invisible SPF 50+, and a velour sponge like the Microfibre Velvet Sponge by JUNO & Co. This sponge doesn't absorb as much as a Beautyblender sponge and so your precious sun protection ends up on your face where it belongs, not in the sponge or the air.

UV filters

Ever wondered why sunscreens are categorised as 'mineral' or 'chemical'? I certainly have. Language is important. As a scientist, I prefer to refer to them as 'inorganic' (mineral) or 'organic' (chemical), because the word 'chemical' has some unfairly negative connotations.

The chemistry term for mineral sunscreen filters is 'inorganic', which refers to a compound that's not carbon-based. In contrast, 'organic' refers to a substance with carbon–hydrogen bonds. Our bodies contain myriad organic compounds.

But it's a false dichotomy, anyway. Both organic and inorganic sunscreens absorb UV radiation and, in doing so, protect our skin.

Inorganic filters

There are two inorganic/mineral UV filters: zinc oxide and titanium dioxide. Both are a white powder in raw form and both absorb UVB and some UVA radiation, with zinc oxide absorbing a wider spectrum of UVA.

They can be difficult to formulate into a pleasant feeling and looking sunscreen formula and are usually responsible for the dreaded white, grey or purple tinge to your skin. This can be avoided by adding other flesh-toned pigments to the formula, which brings its own set of challenges – people come in many different skin tones and all skin needs sunscreen.

Inorganic UV filters are also responsible for the dry, paste-like texture of many sunscreens, and can sometimes give off a metallic scent throughout the day. They may be less likely to slide around your face and into your eyes, but it's all in the formula.

Organic filters

There are nearly 30 organic/chemical filters approved for use in Australia (I love a blend). Most organic UV filters are lipophilic, meaning they dissolve better in oil than water or they're oily liquids themselves. This means they can feel moisturising but sometimes greasy. A good blend of organic filters can give your skin very high sun protection, but again, it's all in the formula.

Inorganic vs organic filters

There are a few reasons people seek out inorganic UV filters in particular, and a lot of the time we're led to believe they're the safer option. I disagree.

There's a widespread belief that inorganic UV filters reflect UV, while organic UV filters absorb and convert to heat. This is not the full story. In fact, all kinds of UV filters mostly absorb and convert to heat, and the heat generated is negligible. Inorganic filters do reflect a little UV, but no more than 15%. There are also some organic UV filters that reflect a little UV radiation.

Which sunscreen is right for you?

It's subjective. You need to think about your skin and lifestyle needs and take it from there. Are you experiencing hyperpigmentation or sensitivity? Then you'll want the highest protection possible, from UVA to UVB, because UV radiation makes hyperpigmentation and sensitivity worse. Do you prefer a glow or more of a mattifying effect? Somewhere in between? Do you like a scent? Do you need your sunscreen to be sweat-resistant for exercise? Or water-resistant for swims? Do you prefer all-in-ones? Or do you want a separate moisturiser and sunscreen? I've reviewed so, so many sunscreens and compiled a list of my favourites for you.

At the end of the day, an SPF 30 you love wearing daily will always be a better option than an SPF 50+ you hate and avoid.

If you're up for it, Google image search 'truck driver sun damage'. You'll find an image of a man that drove a truck for 28 years. On his driver's side, the photodamage has progressed much further – that's UVA damage, through a window! This is why you still need to wear sunscreen indoors.

SUNSCREEN

MY FAVOURITE SUNSCREENS

For a matte finish

— Cancer Council SPF 50+ Face Day Wear Moisturiser Invisible
(Australia only)

For a satin finish

— La Roche-Posay Anthelios Invisible SPF 50+ (AU/UK)
— La Roche-Posay Anthelios Ultra-Light Fluid Face Sunscreen
SPF 60 (US)
— SkinCeuticals Ultra Facial Defense SPF 50+ (AU/UK)

For a glow

— Ultra Violette Queen Screen SPF 50+ (AU/UK)
— Neutrogena Hydro Boost Water Gel Lotion Sunscreen
SPF 50+ (AU/UK/US)

My ultimate SPF is the ISDIN Eryfotona AK-NMSC SPF 100+
Fluid, a European sunscreen. I like very high SPF sunscreens
because I live in Australia and the sun is punishing. This one
was designed to be extremely protective for people with
precancerous changes to their skin.

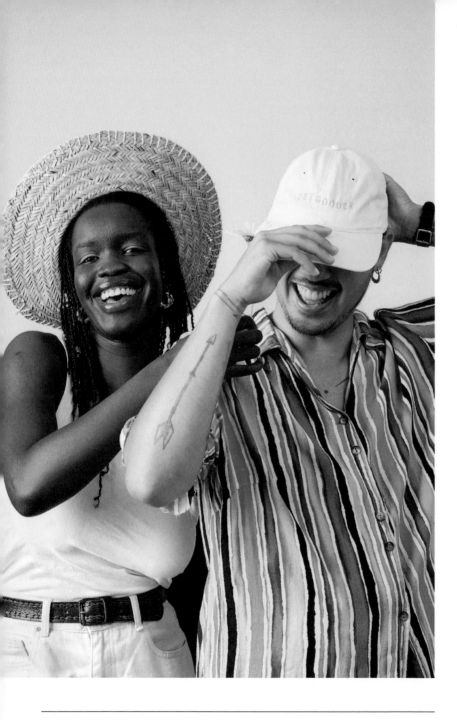

SUNSCREEN

Key takeaways

— Wear sunscreen daily and make it a habit like brushing your teeth. Your skin will thank you.

— Don't forget to put sunscreen on your hands, neck and chest, and inside/behind your ears.

— Sunscreen is only one part of sun-safe behaviour. Get a good-quality hat and sunglasses. It's an investment in your skin.

— Apply a lot of sunscreen – a ½ teaspoon for your face, neck and ears, and 1 teaspoon for each limb. Use a measuring scoop if needed.

— The higher the SPF, the better.

— The best sunscreen is the one you'll wear.

Cleansing

[CHAPTER 6]

Cleansing is potentially the most challenging step for your skin. You do it often, it can rearrange or even remove your barrier lipids, and there's lots of rubbing (potential exfoliation and agitation). That's not to say don't do it – you definitely should – but choose the gentlest cleanser you possibly can for your skin's needs. Mild cleansing can help reduce symptoms of eczema, acne and rosacea. If your skin is prone to hyperpigmentation that is related to inflammation, cleansing gently and keeping the barrier intact can also help prevent further dark spots.

Why do you need to cleanse?

Let's start with the basics. I want to talk about why we need to wash our faces because many of us operate under a lot of assumptions that aren't always correct. Here's a run-down of what we're actually washing off our faces and why it's important.

COMPOUND	WHAT IS IT?	WHY DO WE NEED TO WASH IT OFF?
Sebum	Your skin's 'oil', made up of waxes, triglycerides, free fatty acids and squalene	Excess sebum can form a plug in the pore
Eccrine sweat	Water, salts, ammonia, urea, lactic acid	Bacteria eat these and grow, giving off a scent
Apocrine sweat	Water, sulphur, lipids, steroids, pheromones	Bacteria eat these and grow, giving off a scent
Dead skin cells	Cornified keratinocytes that come loose every day	Excess or build-up can clog the pore
Makeup/ sunscreen	Products containing polymers that form a film on your face	Traps in oil, dead skin cells and sweat over time
Environmental stresses	Dust, air pollution/ smog, airborne irritants	These are sticky and can stress your skin out, leading to inflammation
Microbes	Microorganisms living on and in your skin	While a diverse microbiome is great, touching your face introduces a lot of bacteria

It's not that your skin is dirty, it's just that all this stuff accumulates and it's important to clean it off regularly. Your skin has a natural film of sweat and oil that traps and accumulates a build-up of dust, air pollution, cigarette smoke and whatever else is in the air, on top of anything you've applied that day.

Air pollution molecules are particularly nasty – they're sticky and love to sit in the oils on your skin. Cleansing them off is important for long-term skin health so they don't wreak havoc. It's also beneficial to use skincare that forms a protective film to prevent the molecules from penetrating further – when a skincare product says 'anti-pollution', that's usually what it's referring to.

Loose dead skin cells will also sit on your skin after exfoliation (either naturally, mechanically or chemically) until you wash your face.

What is a cleanser and how does it work?

Cleansers, face washes and body washes remove build-up from your skin and leave behind natural moisturising factor, barrier lipids and good bacteria. The ingredient class that does the cleansing is called a surfactant.

You know how oil kind of floats on the water in a pan until you add detergent? That's what a surfactant does. Surfactants are molecules that interact with both oily things and water, to pick up the build-up on your skin and break it up into something more easily washed away. This is why using an actual cleanser is important. If you just use an oil, it will pick things up from your skin but it won't interact with water for removal. And if you just use water, it won't pick up everything from your skin. You also wouldn't wash your face with dishwashing liquid (although I've tried some cleansers that have felt like it). You need a formula that is gentle for your skin.

On pH

Skin has an acidic pH, which helps to control the bad bacteria on its surface. Your natural oils and sweat help to maintain the pH balance so it makes sense to use a cleanser (and other skincare products) that reflects and respects your natural pH. If pH is too

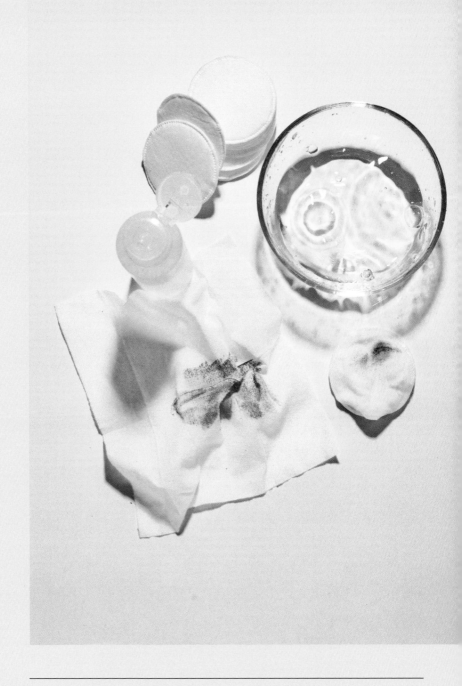

Does your skin feel tight after cleansing? That's not a good thing. It means your cleanser might have got in too far and warped important lipids and proteins. This is usually a good indicator that the cleanser may dry your skin out over the long term.

CLEANSING

high then your barrier can destabilise, proteins can warp and the bad bacteria will throw a party. The pH of water is neutral, so a cleanser should have a pH of 7 or lower. But pH alone doesn't make a cleanser mild – it also depends on the intensity of the surfactants.

It's difficult to find out the pH of a cleanser because this information is not usually listed on the label. Some products will say 'pH balanced', which is a good indicator of a pH that is safe for skin, but this isn't regulated. A useful shortcut is to see if your skin feels tight and dry after cleansing. If it does then you might want to try another product. Avoid using soap as it has too high of a pH for facial cleansing and can be drying. The reason for this is that soap molecules are very good at binding to protein molecules. This isn't ideal as your skin needs those proteins and you don't want them to be washed away or damaged when cleansing. Soap molecules are also similar enough to the lipids in our skin's barrier (e.g. ceramides, cholesterol, free fatty acids) that it can disrupt them. And disrupted barrier lipids means a compromised barrier with faster water loss, faster loss of NMF, and eventually dry, cracked, vulnerable skin.

What about makeup removal wipes?

Even at the height of my insomnia, I never had the energy to do a proper cleanse at night. I used baby wipes and thought I was doing right by my skin as they were fragrance-free and alcohol-free. *Wrong.*

Makeup removal wipes are the worst. I know they're portable and easy but they're not great for your skin. Sorry!

Some wipes contain surfactants (some don't and just move the build-up around on your face where it can contribute to clogged pores), which aren't a great thing to leave on your skin as they're designed to help dissolve oils – and your skin needs some of its oils. Then there's the friction caused by the wipe itself. Wipes can mildly exfoliate, causing redness and slight inflammation, and compromise the barrier. And for some, inflammation contributes to hyperpigmentation.

My suggestion is to say goodbye to your makeup wipes and switch to Bioderma micellar water and a cotton pad. Bioderma makes one for breakout-prone skin and a fragrance-free one for sensitive skin. I promise you'll see an improvement. I keep a bottle on my bedside, with the cotton pads in a fancy jar next to it for the nights I can't manage a full routine.

Categories of cleanser

There are many different types of cleansers in the market. I've broken down the benefits and things to be mindful of for each one.

CATEGORY	GOOD FOR ...	LOOK OUT FOR ...
Oil or balm	Fast, gentle makeup removal; first cleanse	Can clog pores if it leaves a film
Exfoliating (powder, enzyme, acid)	Post-workout; pre-treatment; second or morning cleanse; preventing clogged pores	Over-exfoliation
Micellar water	Quick, easy, rinse-free; first or morning cleanse	Some are too harsh to be left on skin
Gel or foaming	Removal of excess oil; second or morning cleanse	Dehydration
Milk/cream	Any skin type, especially dry skin; first, second or morning cleanse	Residue
Clay	Removal of excess oil; second or morning cleanse	Dehydration

MY FAVOURITE CLEANSERS

— Elemis AHA Glow Cleansing Butter
— MUJI Oil Cleanser
— Frank Body Anti-Makeup Cleansing Oil
— HoliFrog Shasta AHA Refining Acid Wash
— La Roche-Posay Effaclar Micro-Peeling Cleanser
— CeraVe SA Smoothing Cleanser
— Skinstitut L-Lactic Cleanser
— Bioderma Sensibio H2O Micellar Water
— Fresh Soy Face Cleanser
— Skinstitut Gentle Cleanser
— Stratia Skin Velvet Cleansing Milk
— Avène Extremely Gentle Cleanser Lotion
— Biologique Recherche Lait VIP O2
— CeraVe Hydrating Cream to Foam Cleanser
— NIOD Sanskrit Saponins
— REN Clearcalm Clay Cleanser
— Sodashi Clay Cleanser with Sandalwood

QUIZ: WHAT'S THE RIGHT CLEANSER FOR YOU?

Take this quiz to find the right cleanser for you. I like to have a few different cleansers on hand depending on what my skin needs at the time.

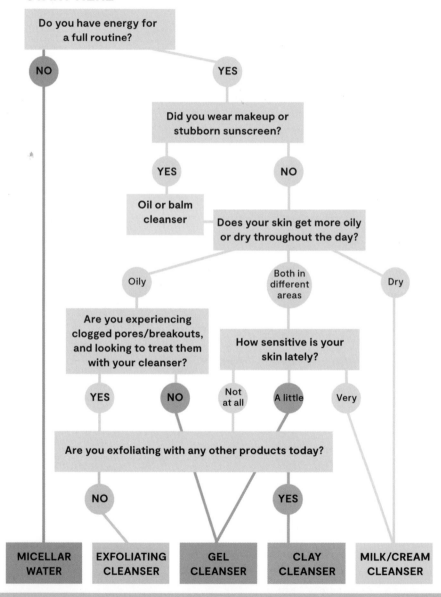

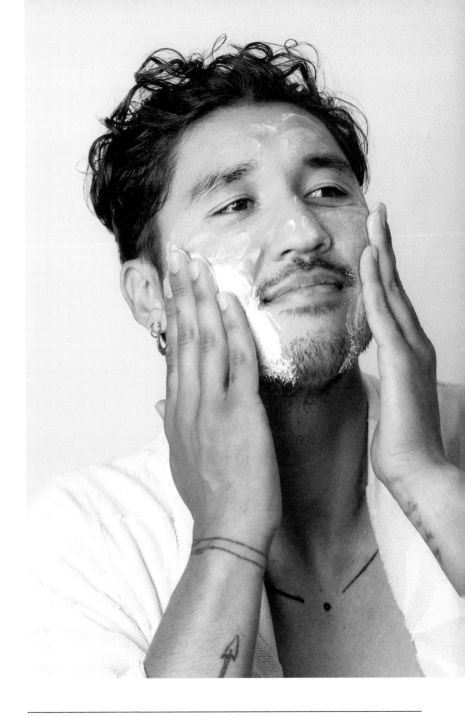

Your cleansing routine

The morning cleanse – do I have to?

If you're someone with sensitive or dry skin, you can probably get away with a mist or splash of water in the morning. If you're more oily, tend to sweat in the night, do morning workouts or are prone to clogged pores, you'll probably need to cleanse in the morning as well. Personally, I need a morning cleanse in summer but am likely to skip the morning cleanse in winter.

The evening cleanse – how to do it properly

To remove all the unwanted stuff (nasty smog and excess dead skin and sebum) and keep the good stuff (NMF, barrier lipids), you need to clean your skin in the gentlest yet most thorough way possible.

I recommend a double cleanse. The first cleanse removes the pollution, makeup and build-up throughout the day; and the second cleanse treats your skin concerns. You can use the same or two different cleansers. If you do a single cleanse, take your time and make sure to be thorough.

Cleansing properly makes a huge difference to the look and feel of your skin. Massage gently, taking your time to cover every area, and make sure to rinse away all of the cleanser. I see a build-up of clogged pores in areas I miss, such as the temples and between the brows.

Now, if you haven't experienced the pure, unadulterated joy that is applying an oil cleanser onto dry skin at the end of the day and watching your makeup come right off … then I have a treat for you. Oil cleansing works on the chemistry principle that like dissolves like. Oil-based substances often dissolve any films and excess oils on your skin (and the oily molecules from smog that are hanging out in there) more easily than water-based cleansers – and with little to no scrubbing.

Here's what you do:

1. Wash your hands and apply the oil cleanser to a dry face.

2. Wet your hands and add warm water to your face to 'emulsify'. This is where the surfactant in the oil cleanser interacts with water.

3. Spend 30 seconds massaging the cleanser into your skin, then remove with water or the softest washcloth you can find. This is your makeup removal step.

4. Use your second cleanser to get into your skin and target your skin concerns, any residual excess oil, leftover oil cleanser and dead skin yet to be rinsed away. Spend at least 30 seconds on this step to ensure you haven't missed any spots (more sensitive skin might require less time).

If you're not using an oil cleanser, here are the steps to follow:

1. Wash your hands.

2. Apply cleanser to damp hands and lather.

3. Apply lather to dry face and work in for 30 seconds, adding more water as you go.

4. Remove with water or a soft washcloth.

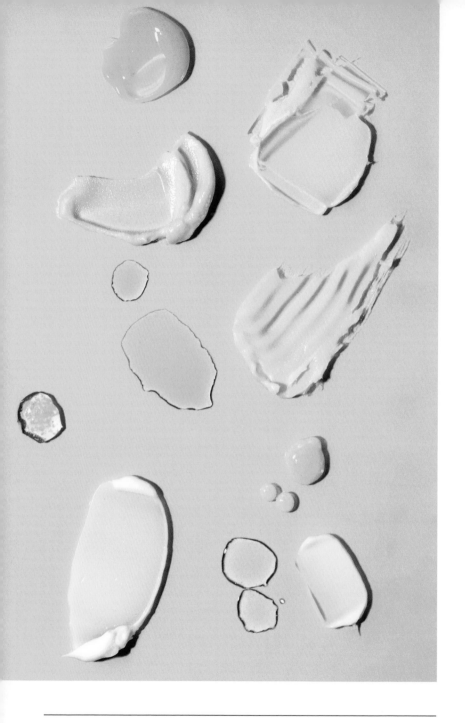

CLEANSING

Key takeaways

— Cleansing is the make-or-break step of your routine.

— There are different cleansers for any skin situation. Cleanse as thoroughly as possible, using the gentlest cleanser you can for your skin's needs.

— Do a double cleanse if you can. The first cleanse removes makeup and build-up and the second cleanse treats your skin concerns.

— Morning cleanses are optional depending on what your skin is doing at the time.

— Makeup wipes are a no-no.

Hydration

[CHAPTER 7]

Picture this: it's winter. Your skin feels tight or dry, or your makeup won't sit right and looks flaky. You put on the thickest moisturiser you can find to fix it. But it just makes your skin feel heavy and greasy. Or your skin still wants more.

Picture another scenario: it's summer this time. Even though a natural glow is beautiful, you don't want your skin to look oily. So you don't moisturise. It's heavy! And it could make you break out.

Knowing the right moisturiser to use can be hard. But all skin needs to stay hydrated – even skin that is prone to breakouts. Let's look at how you can choose the right moisturiser to suit your skin's needs.

—

Hydrating vs moisturising: Medically speaking they're no different – the result is the same.

Keeping your skin hydrated

There are many reasons to keep skin hydrated:

— Water helps your skin feel flexible and moisturised skin looks smooth and bouncy.
— Hydration reduces the appearance of fine lines.
— Water is necessary for a lot of biological processes in your skin, such as making support proteins (e.g. collagen and elastin).
— Moisturising helps the upper layers of skin to stay organised, keeping the environment out and the all-important water in.
— If you're prone to breakouts, hydration helps to keep acne bacteria under control by keeping the barrier sealed.
— Hydrated skin heals better from wounds such as acne lesions. Hydration can even help to reduce potential for scarring.
— Hydrated skin sheds in a more efficient and uniform manner, reducing the chances of dead skin build-up, clogged pores and/or a rough, flaky appearance.

Can moisturisers clog pores?

When you have active acne, it might feel like everything is making you break out. But, in fact, you're breaking out because you have active acne. Acne lesions take 1–2 weeks to form, so you might have one cooking up right now under your skin that will appear in a week's time. There are four main contributing factors to breakouts: inflammation, clogged pores, acne bacteria and individual oil chemistry. Everything else is a factor in these four.

A moisturiser that's too thick might trap dead skin cells and lead to clogged pores in the same way that masks can give us 'mask-ne'. To combat this, look for 'oil-free' on the label, cleanse regularly and thoroughly, and seek the right acne treatment.

Hydrating ingredients

There are three categories of hydrating ingredients: humectants, emollients and occlusives. Some ingredients fall under more than one of these categories, depending on the concentration and formula.

Humectants

Humectants are molecules or substances that **attract water**. They attract water *to* the skin's epidermis *from* the dermis, and act like a sponge, swelling as they collect water and plumping the skin. Humectants that are naturally present in your skin include glycerin (aka glycerol), hyaluronic acid, amino acids, urea, PCA, and even collagen.

Emollients

Emollients are substances that **soften**. They help your skin look and feel smooth and are usually oils or waxes (i.e. lipids). As lipids repel water, they help to keep water in your skin. Their purpose is to sit in place of any missing natural barrier lipids between the cells of your epidermis, which works to keep water in. Some emollients that are naturally present in the skin include cholesterol, squalene (in our sebum) and ceramides.

Occlusives

Occlusives form a **water-repelling barrier**, to push that all-important water back into the skin. The barrier created will prevent your skincare underneath from evaporating, helping it to better absorb. It's not an impermeable barrier but it will dramatically reduce water loss. The level of occlusion will depend on the concentration and other ingredients in a product. Occlusives won't block the movement of water or other substances completely. Some examples include dimethicone (depending on how it's used), petrolatum, mineral oil, carnauba wax and lanolin – think Vaseline.

—

The reason that sheet masks work so well is due to occlusion. The liquid serum can't evaporate because the physical mask is preventing it from doing so.

Moisturisers can be water-based or oil-based. A good moisturiser will contain ingredients from more than one category of hydrating ingredients. If it only uses emollients or occlusives, your skin might look slick but feel tight. Because these ingredients don't work to attract water into the epidermis, they just slow the loss of what's already in there. And if there's not much in there, humectants will help. But if a moisturiser only uses humectants, more water would evaporate. This is why some gel moisturisers can dry you out.

We're not just *adding* water to our skin, we're also helping our skin to *retain* it. The part of our skin that we see (epidermis) gets most of its water from the lower layers of skin – kind of like a limitless source of water.

Choosing the right moisturiser

Choosing the right moisturiser takes a lot of trial and error, but ask yourself the following questions to help you get started:

— *Is my skin dry right now?* Look for emollients and occlusives. Dehydrated? Look for humectants. Both? Look for all three!
— *Do some creams feel too heavy?* If so, look for something lightweight with more humectants than emollients.
— *Do I have clogged pores or am I afraid of getting clogged pores?* If so, look for a moisturiser labelled 'oil-free'.
— *Is my barrier impaired? Am I flaky and sensitive?* If so, look for an occlusive to act in place of the barrier while it regenerates.
— *What time of year is it?* In summer, skin is oilier but still needs hydration; in winter, skin is drier. You might need a lightweight texture in summer but a heavier cream in winter.
— *How humid is it?* Indoor heating and air conditioning can dehydrate your skin as they dry out the air. You may find adding extra emollients or a face oil can help.

—

Dry vs dehydrated skin: Dry skin needs more oils, while dehydrated skin needs more water. Many people experience both, and the answer is the same — moisturise.

Dehydrated skin

Have you ever applied the thickest cream on your face, hoping to help out your dry skin, only to find that it's still tight or flaky? Your skin is probably dehydrated, not dry. And dehydrated skin needs more water. Choose a moisturiser or serum with lots of humectants and some emollients. Try applying it to damp skin, to trap that water.

Dry skin

If your skin is truly dry – eczema-prone, postmenopausal or consistently itchy – then it isn't making enough oil and barrier lipids. This skin type is relatively uncommon before menopause. Using an emollient-rich moisturiser is a solid strategy to address dry skin.

Don't scrub your skin if it is rough, dry and flaky. Hydrate instead and help your skin to shed naturally. Hydrated skin sheds better, whereas scrubbing will continually challenge your barrier, making it harder for skin to stay hydrated and feeding the cycle of dryness.

Oily skin

If you've always seen your skin as oily, you might be trying to reduce oil and shine. Use products that don't feel heavy, sticky or sweaty and won't clog pores. Look for 'oil-free' on the label and for moisturisers rich in humectants.

There are some worked examples in Chapter 9, which show you how to read an ingredient list.

Moisturising product types

Here's a guide to moisturising product types in order of increasing physical thickness (or viscosity).

PRODUCT TYPE	WHAT IS IT?	GOOD FOR ...
Mist/toner	A face mist is a toner but in convenient mist packaging	Easily making your skin damp, to better absorb other products; delivering moisture without feeling heavy
Essence	Usually contains fermented ingredients	Hydrating with brightening benefits for those prone to hyperpigmentation
Serum	A concentrated, water-based way to deliver active ingredients	Gradually improving your skin's capability to moisturise itself
Sheet mask	A huge dose of serum in a sachet with a mask included	Prepping your skin for a special occasion, or use after a procedure
Face oil	Quite liquid and packed with emollients	Sealing in extra moisture for very dry skin or in the winter
Moisturiser	Usually a mix of oil and water; ranges from water gel to a thick cream; thickness is not an indicator of moisturising efficacy	Those after a simple skincare routine (the right moisturiser can be a one-step skincare routine – aside from cleansing and sunscreen)

PRODUCT TYPE	WHAT IS IT?	GOOD FOR ...
<u>Sunscreen</u>	Usually a lotion, which can also act as a moisturiser for daytime	Sun protection and hydration in the one step
<u>Ointment/balm</u>	Thickest	Acting as a replacement barrier when yours is compromised

What if a moisturiser isn't enough?

If you still feel dry or tight after applying a moisturiser, here are some other strategies to try.

Apply moisturiser to damp skin

This is very simple and it makes a world of difference. Try it on both face and body.

The hydration sandwich

This is my AM skincare routine if I need to quickly sort out dehydration issues – maybe my makeup is looking dry and flaky or separating on my face. It's also the routine I use when doing someone else's makeup.

1. Cleanse using a cleanser that leaves your skin soft, not tight. (Or don't cleanse, if your skin is very dry, dehydrated or sensitive, or if you feel like your skin needs a break.)

2. Mist your face, leave it damp from cleansing, or press in a hydrating toner or essence. Use a skincare mist, such as the Evian/La Roche-Posay/Avène Spring Water mists, or put filtered water in a mist bottle.

3. Apply a hydrating serum to your skin while it's damp. This way, you're giving the humectants in the serum some water to take with it into your skin.

4. Add a couple drops of face oil to your moisturiser and let the moisturiser sink in to your skin.

5. Apply sunscreen. I reach for oilier or creamier sunscreens in winter when my skin is more dry. Let it settle on your skin for a minute.

6. If you're wearing makeup, consider adding a hydrating primer to particularly dehydrated areas. For me, that's around my chin, the corners of my mouth, and sometimes my cheeks.

The 7 Skin Method

For this method, 'Skin' refers to a hydrating toner, so what you do is apply up to seven (yes, seven!) layers of your chosen hydrating toner. Do at least two or three layers as it helps to plump out your skin and won't feel heavy at all.

This is a great method if you want to limit the number of products or steps in your skincare routine. It's also great for those prone to sensitivity or rosacea because using fewer products will reduce the chances of a product causing issues.

Key takeaways

— Skin needs to stay hydrated, even if you're prone to breakouts.

— Humectants are great for all skin conditions, climates and situations.

— Lightweight emollients are great for hot weather and/or oily areas of your skin.

— Thicker emollients and occlusives are great for winter and/or drier skin.

— At the end of the day, the best moisturising product is the one that works for you and makes you feel comfortable.

Exfoliation

Skin sheds all the time. It's doing it now. If it's not shedding properly, it can leave your skin looking rough or flaky, or clog your pores and result in breakouts. Hydrated skin is better at shedding, and if you're sure your skin is hydrated enough, this is when you might choose to help it along with exfoliation.

Do you need to exfoliate?

Not everyone needs to incorporate exfoliation into their skincare routine, but here are some reasons why you might choose to:

— You are prone to breakouts or have clogged pores.
— You have hyperpigmentation you wish to help clear.
— You have keratosis pilaris (a condition that causes rough patches and small hard bumps on the skin, often on the backs of arms).
— You want your skin to look smoother.
— You're going to use a treatment product and want it to absorb well (advanced skincare users only).

Exfoliation can also be targeted. For example, I get clogged pores on my nose and I target the area by using an acid toner only on my nose, leaving my sensitive cheeks well alone.

Methods of exfoliation

Mechanical exfoliation

Mechanical exfoliation involves using physical force to remove dead skin cells. This occurs to a small extent during your usual cleansing or it can be done with a washcloth, physical scrub, polishing powder cleanser or cleansing brush/device. It's not a very precise process. There is no need to be aggressive when scrubbing with a product, device or washcloth – the exfoliation happens at a microscopic level and too much pressure will irritate your skin. Never do this on broken or inflamed skin.

Chemical exfoliation

Chemical exfoliation involves using skincare ingredients to normalise cell turnover by influencing living cells and/or selectively dissolving the bonds between the upper (dead) layers of cells. Each exfoliating ingredient has different benefits and combining them can target different skin concerns. Call it synergy. You *must* use sunscreen daily for a week after using a chemical exfoliant as it can make your skin more vulnerable to the sun's damaging effects.

In-clinic chemical peels are also a type of chemical exfoliation, only these are much stronger, hence the need for a licence or medical supervision to complete these treatments.

—

As we age, the skin's turnover slows down. Using exfoliating products helps to remove the dead cells and stimulate them to turn over more quickly like they used to.

Types of exfoliants

TYPE OF EXFOLIANT	GOOD FOR ...	LOOK OUT FOR ...
Washcloth	Removing makeup, SPF, cleanser	Can irritate if too scratchy
Cleansing device	Areas prone to build-up and clogged pores	Overdoing it, scrubbing too hard
Exfoliating cleanser	Gentle use (gentler than a leave-on)	Can be too much for daily use
Physical scrub	Non-inflamed breakouts only	Aggravating inflamed skin
Acid toner	Lightweight, quick exfoliation	Can be quite strong
Acid serum	Gentle use (gentler than a toner)	Potential to overdo it so introduce it slowly
Spot treatment	Treating specific areas	Treats symptoms, not the cause
Exfoliating lotion	Body care	Over-exfoliation if using as a daily moisturiser
Mask	Less frequent use, event preparation	Can be messy, time-consuming

—

There are many types of exfoliants available, but you should tread lightly. I'd use one to two max.

MY FAVOURITE EXFOLIANT PRODUCTS

— Press Beauty Swipies
— MakeUp Eraser
— Skin Gym Swipey Makeup Remover Towel
— FOREO LUNA Mini 3
— HoliFrog Shasta AHA Refining Wash
— African Botanics Buchu Botanical Enzyme Polish
— Biologique Recherche Lotion P50W
— Paula's Choice RESIST Advanced Smoothing Treatment
— REN AHA Smart Renewal Body Serum
— Frank Body Smoothing AHA Body Lotion
— Juice Beauty Green Apple Peel
— Versed Doctor's Visit Instant Resurfacing Mask

Exfoliating ingredients

Don't fixate on the percentage of exfoliating acid in a product – it isn't the only factor. The strength also depends on which acid(s) the product contains and its pH. Two different products with the same percentage of glycolic acid can feel wildly different on the skin, so always observe your skin and how it responds to exfoliating products.

AHAs

Daily use of AHAs (alpha hydroxy acids) can help improve hydration, thicken and normalise the dermis and epidermis, improve the quality of collagen, improve barrier function and even stimulate fibroblasts to make more collagen. You MUST wear sunscreen for a week after using AHAs as they increase sensitivity to the sun. AHAs are characteristically water-soluble and often found in products for 'aged', dry or sun-damaged skin – they're also now popping up more in acne products. (They've helped me a lot with my acne too.)

BHAs

Unlike AHAs, BHAs (beta hydroxy acids) do not increase sun sensitivity. They are oil-soluble, meaning they're particularly useful in oily areas, exfoliating inside the pores as well as on the surface.

PHAs

PHAs (or polyhydroxy acids) are very hydrating and gentler than AHAs, so they're safe to use even on sensitive or rosacea-prone skin. They don't sting nor increase UV sensitivity. They're also anti-glycation (see Glossary).

Exfoliating enzymes

Exfoliating enzymes break down proteins, such as the keratin in the top layers of corneocytes. You might feel a tingle from them, but they're gentler than scrubs and an alternative option to using acids. Bear in mind that enzymes are unstable so you need to store your enzyme products as instructed.

I've listed some commonly used exfoliating ingredients below and how you might use them.

INGREDIENT	WHAT IS IT?	WHAT DOES IT DO?
AHAs		
Glycolic acid	A humectant found naturally in sugar cane and lemons. It is the smallest molecule and so penetrates the deepest.	Because glycolic acid penetrates deeply, it can cause a tingling sensation and be tricky for sensitive skin or those with rosacea or prone to post-inflammatory hyperpigmentation. It will increase your risk of sun damage and sunburn so you need to wear sunscreen for at least a week after use. Look for 4–10% concentration, with a pH of 3–4.
Lactic acid	A larger molecule, generally gentler. It's found in sour milk and tomatoes, and in your skin's NMF. It's also a humectant.	Can be moisturising and/or exfoliating, depending on the product, pH and concentration. It can also cause tingling and help to support the barrier (if you don't overdo it) by facilitating an increase in ceramides. Look for 5–12% concentration if you want it to exfoliate, and a pH of 3–4.

INGREDIENT	WHAT IS IT?	WHAT DOES IT DO?
Mandelic acid	Found naturally in bitter almond	Great for dry, sensitive, pigmented or acne-prone skin. It's partially oil-soluble, with antibacterial properties, and well tolerated by sensitive skin; look for 5–10% concentration with a pH of 3–4
Malic acid	Comes from apples	Has antioxidant properties and is most useful in a blend
Tartaric acid	Found in fruits such as pomegranate	May help support the barrier and has antioxidant properties
Citric acid	Found in pineapple, lemon and other citrus	Not as effective at encouraging hydration and cell turnover as glycolic or lactic acids; however, it is gentler and has antioxidant properties, and will work alone or in a blend
BHAs		
Salicylic acid	Found naturally in willow bark	Exfoliating and anti-inflammatory, making it a great way to treat acne. Salicylic acid exfoliates from the top layer down; look for 0.5–2% concentration
Willow bark extract	Willow bark (obviously)	Only contains a tiny bit of salicylic acid so it probably won't exfoliate; however, it can be anti-inflammatory

INGREDIENT	WHAT IS IT?	WHAT DOES IT DO?
Betaine salicylate	Similar to salicylic acid	A gentler and moisturising version of salicylic acid – look for 2–4% concentration
Caprylol salicylic acid	Known as LHA (lipohydroxy acid); it's a salicylic acid with a lipid chain attached, making it a bigger molecule	Doesn't penetrate skin as quickly or deeply, so is a gentler oil-soluble exfoliant
PHAs		
Gluconic acid, gluconolactone acid and lactobionic acid	Bigger molecules	Gentle and doesn't increase UV sensitivity. Gluconolactone acid and lactobionic acid are the best researched; look for concentrations around 10%
Exfoliating enzymes		
Papaya, pineapple, and pumpkin	Exfoliating enzymes	Breaks down proteins so you might feel a tingle; look for papaya (papain/*Carica papaya* fruit extract), pineapple (bromelain/ *Ananas sativus* fruit extract) and pumpkin (*Cucurbita pepo*)

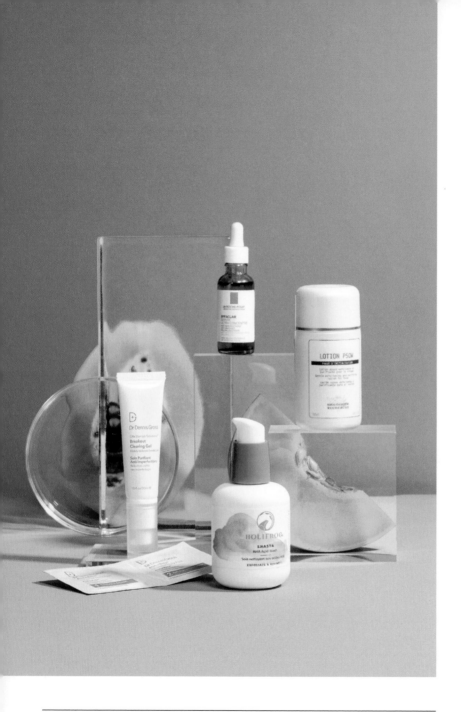

EXFOLIATION

Other chemical exfoliants

INGREDIENT	WHAT IS IT?	WHAT DOES IT DO?
Retinoids	Vitamin A, the gold standard in acne treatment and reversal of sun damage	Retinoids don't break bonds between dead cells, but they do signal skin to normalise cell turnover
Urea	Found naturally in your skin, so it's well tolerated	Urea is hydrating at low concentrations and exfoliates at high concentrations (10%+)
Pyruvic acid	Exists in our bodies as part of cellular respiration; mostly found in professional peels	Exfoliates, reduces oil and is antimicrobial (kills bacteria)
Kojic acid	Comes from the rice fermentation process (making sake)	Lightly exfoliates, but is better known as a potent pigment blocker for treatment of hyperpigmentation
Azelaic acid	Found in grains, such as barley	A great ingredient best used at 10–20% concentration. It's not really an exfoliant but it does influence the way cells mature and shed, helping to prevent clogged pores. It's also mildly antimicrobial and helps reduce inflammation, so it's great for rosacea and acne, plus it's very effective for some types of hyperpigmentation; you might need a prescription in some countries

Choosing the right exfoliant

Sometimes the instructions on skincare products are a little *irresponsible*. For example, when I was younger I purchased a BHA exfoliant that said to 'use once to twice daily' … so I did. It made my acne worse within days because that was way too much BHA for me. It's a good idea to incorporate an exfoliant into your routine slowly – once to twice per week for a couple of weeks, then increase to every second day if you need to, as tolerated. Your problems will not resolve any faster by using exfoliants too often, too soon. What it will do is exacerbate them and then put you off using exfoliants at all.

Exfoliating does show some immediate benefits, such as smoother-looking skin, but the best results can take up to four weeks, and even as long as six months, depending on the product, the rest of your skincare routine, and your skin's condition and needs. The only way to speed that up is with a time machine, so take it easy.

Tingling is not necessarily a bad thing, but it can be an indicator that your skin can't take much more. However, you can still overdo it without feeling a tingling sensation.

Many products combine one or more exfoliating ingredients and/or methods. Some cleansers exfoliate both mechanically with grains and chemically with enzymes, and some masks combine enzymes and acids.

When choosing an exfoliant, ask yourself these questions:

— *Do I need to exfoliate?* Is there something else in your skincare routine that could do the same thing? For example, after a long, sweaty day, might a clay mask be a gentler option to unclog pores?
— *Could my skin issue be resolved through more hydration?* If skin is flaky, exfoliating won't rehydrate skin.
— *Which ingredients are exfoliating ones?* Are these ideal for your skin concerns and goals?

— *How sensitive is my skin?* Should you start with a gentler option? PHAs are perfect for rosacea or sensitive areas.
— *Am I treating hyperpigmentation, acne or textural issues?* See Chapters 11 and 13.
— *Am I after something I can use daily or weekly?* Think about your lifestyle, what you can reasonably commit to and the rest of your skincare routine. Don't push your skin too far. Skincare should be fun, not stressful.

MY FAVOURITE EXFOLIATING PRODUCTS

— HoliFrog Shasta AHA Cleanser: Amazing for post-workout breakout prevention
— Paula's Choice 2% BHA Liquid (toner): Great for targeting clogged pores
— Biologique Recherche Lotion P50W (toner): Gentle yet effective, smells like vinegar, targets clogged pores
— La Roche-Posay Effaclar Serum: For targeting acne and signs of ageing
— Dr Dennis Gross Breakout Clearing Gel (serum/spot treatment): Incredibly effective for preventing breakouts when used regularly on breakout-prone areas (but smells of sulphur)
— Dr Dennis Gross Universal Peel Pads (treatment): Your smoothest skin yet!

How do you know if you've overdone it?

Easy. You'll have a compromised barrier so you might notice some or all of the following:

— innocuous products that didn't use to sting can start to sting
— tingling, itching, burning
— more breakouts, all at once
— skin feels tight but oily
— skin feels tight, dry and potentially flaky.

Stop using your exfoliant immediately and see Chapter 4 for instructions on how to heal your skin.

Key takeaways

— Exfoliation occurs naturally, but you can help it along if you are prone to breakouts, have clogged pores or hyperpigmentation, or want your skin to look smoother.

— Exfoliants can be used to target key areas and exfoliating ingredients can be combined to address different skin concerns.

— Always introduce an exfoliant slowly — once to twice per week for a couple of weeks, then increase to every second day if you need to.

— The best results can take up to four weeks, and even as long as six months, depending on the product, the rest of your skincare routine, and your skin's condition and needs.

How to read a skincare label

[CHAPTER 9]

Do you read the ingredients of your skincare products? I love to, but I'm probably in the minority here. I want to share what I know so you can be better equipped to assess whether or not a product will do what it promises to do.

First of all, I need you to say this out loud: *the dose makes the poison*. Say it again. Out loud. Let's use alcohol as an example – pure ethanol. Alcohol is great for disinfecting at 60–70% concentration and regularly used in clinics before skin-piercing treatments, such as microneedling. If the concentration is higher, the bacteria know to go dormant to protect themselves. If it's lower, it won't be enough to kill them. In skincare, products containing alcohol will be at a concentration much lower than 60–70% and the alcohol is usually there to thin out the formula or to help the formula deliver its ingredients to where they need to go in your skin.

See? The dose makes the poison.

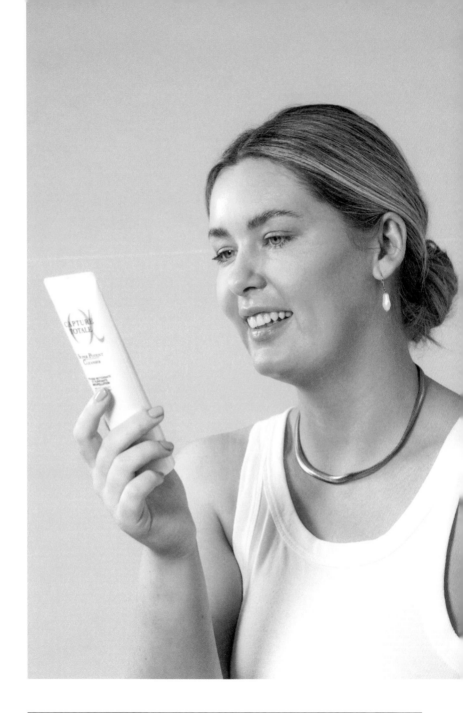

The basics

What you can tell from an ingredients list

— **If it contains specific ingredients that are known to do what the product claims to do.** I'll often scan the active ingredients when investigating a product. For example, if a product claims to 'brighten' skin, I might expect to see vitamin C or niacinamide. If it's for sensitive, compromised skin, I don't like to see lots of fragrant plant oils like lavender or geranium. They're not bad for everyone with sensitive skin, but they make me itchy.

— **Roughly how much of an ingredient is present.** As mentioned before, the dose makes the poison. Some ingredients, such as alcohol, get a bad rap but have their uses. Alcohol is a great penetration enhancer and largely evaporates before it sinks into your skin. It's also found in Dr Dennis Gross's fabled Alpha Beta Peel Pads (good luck prying them from my cold, dead hands). Alcohol can be drying at high concentrations, so you wouldn't want a hydrating product like a moisturiser to be 50% alcohol, but 1% would be fine to help dissolve another ingredient. Use your common sense and best judgement.

— **If it contains allergens or ingredients you don't like.** Check for allergens if you have any allergies or ingredients you don't enjoy for whatever reason much like the ingredient list for food.

What you can't tell from an ingredients list

It's like cake. You can look at the ingredients all you like but you won't know how it tastes until you try it. The same goes for the effects of skincare products.

Ingredients list guidelines

There are guidelines for how ingredients are listed on personal care products.

— They must all be named according to the INCI (International Nomenclature of Cosmetic Ingredients), an international standard that ensures ingredients are called the same thing worldwide. For example, the INCI name for green tea is 'Camellia sinensis leaf extract'.
— Everything must be listed in order of quantity. If it's first on the ingredient list, it is the most abundant ingredient. However, this is not true for South Korean products.
— The top five ingredients make up the majority of the mixture, so you can sometimes get a feel for the texture of the product with only this information.
— Many ingredients are effective at very low concentrations so more does not always mean better. Peptides, for example, are effective at very small concentrations – parts-per-million small!
— Once you get down to 1% or less, ingredients can be listed in any order, so brands will sometimes list the most exciting ingredients first.
— Perfume/parfum/aroma is exempted from listing full ingredients as they're considered a trade secret; however, known irritants do need to be listed.

Once you're across this info, it's about recognising which ingredients do what and that takes time and practice.

Use INCI Decoder (https://incidecoder.com/) to decode ingredient lists. Search for products or photograph/copy and paste ingredient lists to get a breakdown of what the ingredients do. The website also categorises products by ingredient.

Ingredient categories

Here are some common ingredient categories that you might come across in your skincare products.

CATEGORY	WHAT DOES IT DO?
Preservative	Preservatives help to prevent growth of bacteria and mould in products. Some commonly used safe and effective preservatives include phenoxyethanol, methylparaben, potassium sorbate, benzoic acid, chlorphenesin and caprylhydroxamic acid. Some products use sterile packaging instead of preservatives.
Solvent	Solvents are ingredients that dissolve other ingredients. Water is a solvent for sugar or salt. Alcohol is another example of a solvent, as well as propylene glycol which is used in many applications for its moisturising action.
Chelating agent	Chelating agents react with metal ions and prevent them from reacting with our skin or products, to keep things stable. There are metal ions in water (especially hard water, which makes it challenging for skin and hair) and other skincare ingredients such as iron oxide pigments. Metal ions can sometimes help bacteria to grow so chelating agents can make preservatives work better.
Buffer	Buffers are used to adjust the pH of skincare products. For example, it can ensure a moisturiser is not too acidic.

CATEGORY	WHAT DOES IT DO?
Surfactant	Surfactants break surface tension. They enable oil and water to mix in order to cleanse oil from skin, create a foam, make lipids and water-soluble ingredients sit nicely in a moisturiser without separating, and help deliver ingredients into your skin. Some are kinder to skin than others.
Emulsifier	An emulsifier is a type of surfactant that helps mix things together that wouldn't otherwise mix. Its job in personal care products is to stabilise the oil and water phases so the product doesn't separate. It's very important that oil and water don't separate, especially in sunscreens, which must form an even film of UV filter to adequately protect skin.

—

If you're having issues with a skincare product, note what's on the ingredient list in case you run into the same issue with another product later. Knowledge is power.

Deciphering the words

Skincare is full of buzzwords so here is a no-nonsense explanation as to what those label claims on your products really mean.

BUZZWORD	WHAT IT REALLY MEANS ...
Sulphate-free	'No SLS' means it does not contain sodium lauryl sulphate, which is an effective surfactant. It's not dangerous but it can be drying for skin and hair if the product isn't formulated with lots of moisturising ingredients. You would expect to find SLS in a product that cleans (e.g. cleanser, shampoo, dishwashing liquid). But if the product says 'sulphate-free' and it's not a product that cleans ... well, that seems a bit silly to me.
Natural	This means some of the ingredients come from natural sources (i.e. minerals or plants) with minimal processing. The thing is, this isn't the most sustainable or effective choice for skin, and 'natural' is not synonymous with 'good for you'. Arsenic is natural, for example.
Oil-free	This means no oils are used in the formula. Those with acne-prone skin are often directed to this type of product, to help avoid clogged pores and further breakouts. Oil-free is a good start, but oil-free products can contain other lipids like waxes and still clog pores. Furthermore, products containing oils can also help balance breakout-prone skin without clogging.

BUZZWORD	WHAT IT REALLY MEANS ...
Non-comedogenic	This means the product is designed not to be too heavy and therefore shouldn't clog pores. However, it's not a regulated term. You can check online if individual ingredients are comedogenic, but this assessment is based on that ingredient alone, which will behave *very* differently in a formula with lots of others.
Cruelty-free	This means the product is not tested on animals or sold in countries that conduct mandatory animal testing. However, almost all ingredients have been animal tested for safety at some point. Many countries have now banned animal testing so that brands may not use recent animal testing data to support their claims.
Vegan	This means there are no animal-derived ingredients in the product. A product can be vegan but not 'cruelty-free'.
Fragrance-free	Fragrance-free means there is no fragrance/aroma/parfum in the ingredients. These products are great if you have sensitive skin and/or have an impaired barrier, but they are not necessary for most people. Skin sensitivity to fragrances is uncommon and when it occurs, it's usually to only a few things, not every scent. A product can be fragrance-free and still smell good. Other ingredients, such as a plant or fruit extract, can be used to mask smells.

BUZZWORD	WHAT IT REALLY MEANS ...
No synthetic fragrance	This means that a fragrance may have been added that has come from plant extracts or plant essential oils, or similar. Advocates of this line of thinking will tell you that natural is better, but frankly that's a logical fallacy. Natural fragrances often contain a higher level of known allergens, whereas something synthetic can be controlled for allergen levels.
Chemical-free	Everything is a chemical – think of the word 'chemical' as a synonym for 'substance' or 'matter'. Anything that exists. 'Chemical-free' is meant to imply that there's nothing harmful in the product, but lucky for us, our governments regularly review ingredients that might be harmful and classify them accordingly.
Essential oils	Essential oils are not to be confused with seed oils from the same plant – the extraction process and end composition are different. Plant seed oils are usually not very fragrant. For example, passionfruit essential oil smells like passionfruit (yum) and may contain citronellol, a fragrant molecule that is potentially irritating for some. Conversely, passionfruit seed oil (also known as *Passiflora edulis* seed oil or maracuja oil) is a lightweight face oil that is safe for acne-prone skin and doesn't really have a scent.

Deciphering the symbols

Have you ever noticed these pictures on your product labels? Here's what some of them mean.

SYMBOL	WHAT IT REALLY MEANS …
12M Period after opening	This is how long the product is stable for after opening. 12 M means 12 months, but you'll see anything from 3 M all the way to 36 M.
Green dot recycling	This is a European program and shows that the company has paid a fee to help cover the cost of recycling the packaging.
Leaping bunny	This means no animal testing was used to develop the product.
PETE HDPE V LDPE PP PS OTHER Recycling	This doesn't necessarily mean that the packaging can be recycled – it just shows the type of plastic that the packaging uses.

Deciphering the claims

Vitamin C

Vitamin C is often heralded as a staple in an AM skincare routine, to help prevent free radical damage and boost your sunscreen – plus it's great for promoting collagen, right?

It might surprise you to find out that the research supporting these functions is largely based on pure vitamin C, which is called L-ascorbic acid on an ingredient list. L-ascorbic acid is quite unstable so it doesn't last that long and it can be hard to tolerate for some skin types (mine included). One workaround is to use more stable derivatives, but these must be converted in the skin to L-ascorbic acid before they work and there's just not the same wealth of research to support their benefits.

For example, if a label says '5% pure vitamin C' and the ingredient list doesn't contain L-ascorbic acid but instead includes a derivative such as sodium ascorbyl phosphate, it's not the same thing and shouldn't claim to have the same benefits. Sometimes products don't even contain a derivative and instead use a plant extract that's 'rich in vitamin C', such as Kakadu plum (the highest known natural source of vitamin C at 3–6%).[29]

If L-ascorbic acid is too strong for you, go for the derivative over the plant extract. Plant extracts aren't as concentrated and are therefore harder to derive a result from.

Retinoids

The same thing happens with retinoid products. The label might say 'vitamin A' or 'retinol', but if you check the ingredient list you might find a less-researched derivative such as retinyl palmitate, retinyl propionate or hydroxypinacolone retinoate, or even a plant oil rich in provitamin A. Rosehip oil, for example, is said to be rich in beta-carotene (provitamin A). Rosehip fruit's flesh is around 0.00395% beta-carotene and rosehip oil contains a maximum of 0.000036% retinoic acid (actual vitamin A). It's easier for skincare companies to put 'retinol' on the label than explain the benefits of the specific ester or plant they're using.

If you see '1% retinol complex' on the label, the *complex* part is a giveaway that something's going on – otherwise, it'd just say '1% retinol'. The product could have 1% of a pre-made raw material that itself is 1% retinol, leaving the finished product with only 0.01% retinol. It's still effective, but definitely a step back if you're used to something stronger.

The percentage is also only one piece of the puzzle – ingredients must also be stable and able to absorb into the right part of your skin, where they elicit their effects.

Deciphering the labels

Let's apply our new-found knowledge by looking at some skincare label examples. Note: Emollients are highlighted, humectants are underlined, occlusives are italic.

Kiehl's Ultra Facial Cream. This cream contains a lot of emollients, but the two most abundant ingredients are glycerin and water, followed by an evaporating silicone and then squalane, which is also lightweight and silky. With this information, I can tell that the cream is a lightweight gel and likely won't leave a heavy feeling. Great for combination or dehydrated skin, but you might need a bit more from your cream in winter, or if you're feeling very dry.

AQUA/WATER, GLYCERIN, CYCLOHEXASILOXANE, SQUALANE, BIS-PEG-18 METHYL ETHER DIMETHYL SILANE, SUCROSE STEREATE, STEARYL ALCOHOL, PEG-8 STEREATE, MYRISTYL MYRISTATE, PENTAERYTHRITYL TETRAETHYLHEXANOATE, PRUNUS ARMENIACA KERNEL OIL/APRICOT KERNEL OIL, PHENOXYETHANOL, PERSEA GRATISSIMA OIL/AVOCADO OIL, GLYCERYL STEREATE, CETYL ALCOHOL, ORYZA SATIVA BRAN OIL/RICE BRAN OIL, OLEA EUROPEA FRUIT OIL/OLIVE FRUIT OIL, CHLORPHENESIN, STEARIC ACID, PALMITIC ACID, DISODIUM EDTA, ACRYLATES/C10-30 ALKYL ACRYLATE CROSSPOLYMER, CARBOMER, PRUNUS AMYGDALUS DULCIS OIL/ SWEET ALMOND OIL, XANTHAN GUM, ETHYLHEXYLGLYCERIN, SODIUM HYDROXIDE, TOCOPHEROL, GLYCINE SOJA OIL/SOYBEAN OIL, PSEUDOALTEROMONAS FERMENT EXTRACT, MYRISTIC ACID, HYDROXYPALMITOYL, SPHINGANINE, BHT, SALICYLIC ACID, CITRIC ACID

Indeed Labs Hydraluron Moisture Jelly. Both emollients in this formula are also humectants, so you can tell this formula is a very lightweight gel. Best suited to those living in humid climates or with truly oily skin.

WATER (AQUA/EAU), GLYCERIN, PENTYLENE GLYCOL, GLYCERETH-26, CARBOMER, GLYCERYL POLYACRYLATE, TREHALOSE, UREA, STRELITZIA NICOLAI SEED ARIL EXTRACT, SODIUM HYDROXIDE, DISODIUM EDTA, SERINE, BIOSACCHARIDE GUM-1, ALGIN, DISODIUM PHOSPHATE, PULLULAN, SODIUM HYALURONATE, POTASSIUM PHOSPHATE, CAPRYLYL GLYCOL, PHENOXYETHANOL

Avène Skin Recovery Cream Rich. From this ingredient list you can tell that the moisturiser is rich. There's mineral oil (a breathable occlusive) and a couple of humectants. As for the emollients, there's squalane, only it's combined with a couple of waxes and shea butter, which is quite thick. It doesn't look like there's *much* shea butter, given it's halfway down the ingredient list, so it's unlikely to clog pores. This moisturiser is a great one for winter or for dry, sensitive skin.

AVENE THERMAL SPRING WATER (AVENE AQUA), *MINERAL OIL (PARAFFINUM LIQUIDUM)*, GLYCERIN, SQUALANE, DIMETHICONE, GLYCERYL STEARATE, BEHENYL ALCOHOL, SERINE, BUTYROSPERMUM PARKII (SHEA) BUTTER, CARBOMER, TETRASODIUM EDTA, TRIETHANOLAMINE, WATER (AQUA), XANTHAN GUM

Key takeaways

— The ingredient list can tell you a lot about a product. Everything must be listed in order of quantity, so if it's first on the ingredient list, it is the most abundant ingredient. Once you get down to 1% or less, ingredients can be listed in any order.

— Many ingredients are effective at very low concentrations, so more does not always mean better. Remember: the dose makes the poison.

— Not all skincare labels and claims are regulated, so make sure you're aware of commonly used buzzwords and symbols and what they really mean.

— You can get an idea of which product will be best for you from the label, but at the end of the day you have to try it, wear it and see how it goes.

Building your skincare routine

[CHAPTER 10]

Let's recap. You now know you need sunscreen and are wearing it daily (this is not optional), you've figured out if you want to treat a specific skin concern or if you just want to keep things happy and healthy, and you know that cleansing gently but thoroughly is a must. So is moisturiser.

Time for the fun part! Let's talk about building your skincare routine.

AM vs PM

During the day, your skin is oilier and most in need of protection from the sun and the environment. At night, skin renews and repairs itself better but is also more prone to water loss. This is why night creams tend to be thicker than day creams.

The best strategy is to protect during the day and hydrate/rebuild at night. Simple, right? A basic routine might look something like this:

— AM: Gentle cleanse, moisturising SPF with antioxidants
— PM: Gentle cleanse, moisturiser

That's three products. Maybe four if you wear makeup, for a double cleanse at night.

We then have to factor in your skin goals. If there's something you want to treat, you might want to look for a treatment night cream or add in a serum or eye cream. If you have more than one skin concern, there's probably a product out there that does it all.

—

Don't forget your neck, chest and the backs of your hands when applying skincare and sunscreen. Your face stops at your nips.

Timeline of changes to skin

AGE	WHAT YOUR SKIN IS DOING	WHAT YOU CAN DO
Childhood	Skin is thinner and more prone to allergy and sun damage regardless of skin tone.	Wear sunscreen and engage in sun-smart behaviour – wear sunglasses, a hat, stay in the shade and wear protective clothing.
Teens	Hormones affect skin by amping up oil production. This is also affected if you're taking androgens to transition.	If needed, introduce a breakout-targeting product (affected areas only) every second day, such as Dr Dennis Gross Breakout Clearing Gel or Paula's Choice BHA Liquid. See a doctor ASAP if breakouts are severe (large, painful lumps under the skin).
Early 20s	Everything is running smoothly but you can still experience breakouts into your 20s and beyond.	Enjoy what you have and keep your skin protected and hydrated.
Late 20s	Cell turnover and collagen and hyaluronic acid production slow down; expression lines and hyperpigmentation start to show.	Add in a hydrating serum and think about introducing a retinoid if you haven't already.

AGE	WHAT YOUR SKIN IS DOING	WHAT YOU CAN DO
30s	The fat under your skin changes, getting thinner in the cheekbone area and thicker around the chin. Sun exposure from earlier in life starts to show up as dilated blood vessels, and damaged and bunched-up collagen and elastin, resulting in a rippled texture, sunspots and wrinkles. Blood vessels and nasolabial folds become more visible and skin needs more moisture. Rosacea often develops from age 30 if you're prone.	If you think you might have rosacea, see a doctor for guidance. Incorporate a pigment blocker if hyperpigmentation is a concern.
40s	Lip lines might appear.	Switch to a richer moisturiser, to replenish lost moisture and natural oils. Switch to lip balm with SPF if you're not using one already.
50s	More facial fat pads are lost and what's left migrates. Menopause happens on average at age 51, and oestrogen-deprived skin is drier, thinner and less elastic (but melasma can resolve due to the same hormonal changes).	Look for richer moisturisers and peptides for firming.
60s+	In your 60s and beyond, dermatologists suggest to shift the focus from skincare to procedures. Skin is rough and sunspots are more prominent. Skincare can help with texture and pigmentation, but it can't replace lost volume.	Keep your skincare simple, moisturising and gentle, as skin can become more sensitive, dry and itchy.

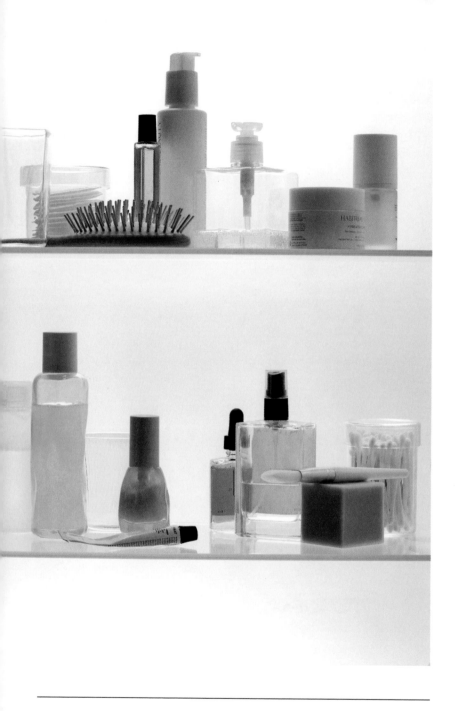

BUILDING YOUR SKINCARE ROUTINE

Basic skincare routines

Here are some suggested skincare routines based on the changes in your skin over the course of your life. You don't have to follow every step – keep it at the bare minimum if that's your preference. Tread lightly with any exfoliants and retinoids, or anything else challenging for your skin (pigment-blocking serums and vitamin C can also feel a little tingly). If you can only tolerate a product once per week, consider switching to another product in that category that is gentle enough for daily use.

AM	PM	WEEKLY	COMMENTS
Childhood			
Cleanser SPF	Cleanser Moisturiser		Kids' skin is more sensitive so find a sunscreen for sensitive skin that your kids like to use.
Teens			
Cleanser SPF	Oil cleanser (if using makeup) Cleanser Moisturiser	Exfoliate 1–3 ×	Skin becomes oilier as you start to see hormonal changes; a targeted exfoliant will work wonders.

AM	PM	WEEKLY	COMMENTS
		20s	
Cleanser Antioxidant serum Moisturising SPF	Oil cleanser (if using makeup) Cleanser Eye cream (optional) Treatment serum (optional) Moisturiser	Exfoliate 1–3 × Mask (optional)	Boost your sunscreen with an antioxidant serum and set yourself up for a bright future.
		30s	
Cleanser Antioxidant serum Moisturiser (optional) SPF	Oil cleanser (if using makeup) Cleanser Eye cream Serum Moisturiser Face oil (optional)	Retinoid 1–2 × Exfoliant 1–2 × Mask (optional)	There are 2-in-1 products that contain retinoids and exfoliants, such as the Skinbetter Science AlphaRet Overnight Cream or the Dr Dennis Gross Ferulic + Retinol Peel. You'll start to need extra hydration and will see benefits from boosting cell turnover.

AM	PM	WEEKLY	COMMENTS
40s			
Cleanser (optional) Antioxidant serum Moisturiser SPF	Oil cleanser (if using makeup) Cleanser Hydrating serum Eye cream (optional) Moisturiser Face oil (optional)	Retinoid 3–4 × Exfoliant/ peel 1+ × (as tolerated)	If your skin is becoming sensitive, skip your morning cleanse (but you can do that at any age, really).
50s+			
Cleanser (optional) Antioxidant serum Eye cream (optional) Moisturiser SPF	Cleanser Eye cream (optional) Hydrating serum Moisturiser Face oil (optional)	Retinoid 4 × Exfoliant/ peel 1+ × (as tolerated)	In-clinic treatments can help if that's something you have the time or budget for.

Order of skincare

For me, the order of skincare products isn't super important and it depends on what you're trying to achieve. Here are some principles to operate on:

1. Thinnest to thickest.

2. Think about which actives (if any) you're using. Do you want them as close to the skin as possible? Or do you want to cushion your skin by applying something else to dilute it first?

3. Eye cream goes on before serum and moisturiser, to help protect the eye area and to ensure it has a chance to soak in.

You've probably been told, 'This ingredient clashes with that or inactivates this'. How exhausting. Too many rules. My advice? Keep your treatment products minimal. Then you'll never run into this problem.

ROUTINE: DAILY SKINCARE

Here's an example skincare routine. You don't have to incorporate every step (in fact, I'd rather you didn't), but if you *were* to use all of these products, this is the suggested order in which you'd use them.

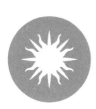

Daily Skincare Routine

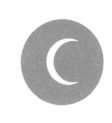

[day]	[night]
CLEANSER	OIL CLEANSE
MASK	SECOND CLEANSE
MIST	MIST
EYE CREAM	EYE CREAM
TONER OR ESSENCE	TONER
SERUM	ESSENCE
FACE OIL	SERUM
MOISTURISER	FACE OIL
SUNSCREEN	MOISTURISER
MAKEUP	SLEEPING MASK/ HEALING BALM
	LIP MASK

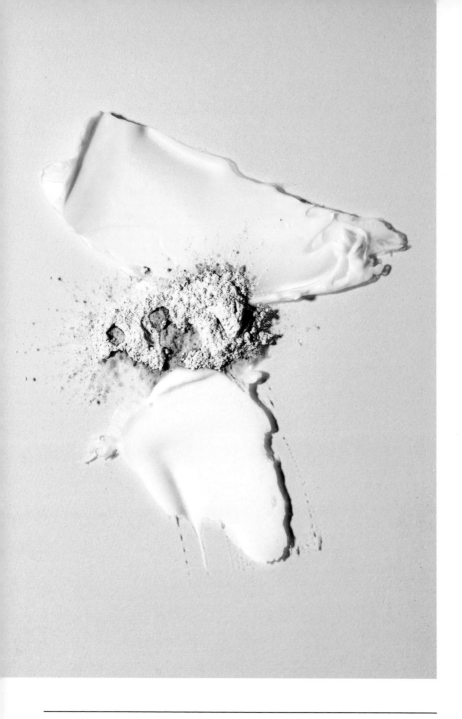

BUILDING YOUR SKINCARE ROUTINE

Key takeaways

— The best strategy to incorporate for your skincare routine is to protect during the day and treat/hydrate/rebuild at night, factoring in your skin goals and concerns.

— You don't have to do all of the steps — keep your skincare routine as basic as you like. Figure out your priorities for your skin and lifestyle.

— Adapt your skincare routine according to the changes in your skin over the course of your life.

Your skin concerns

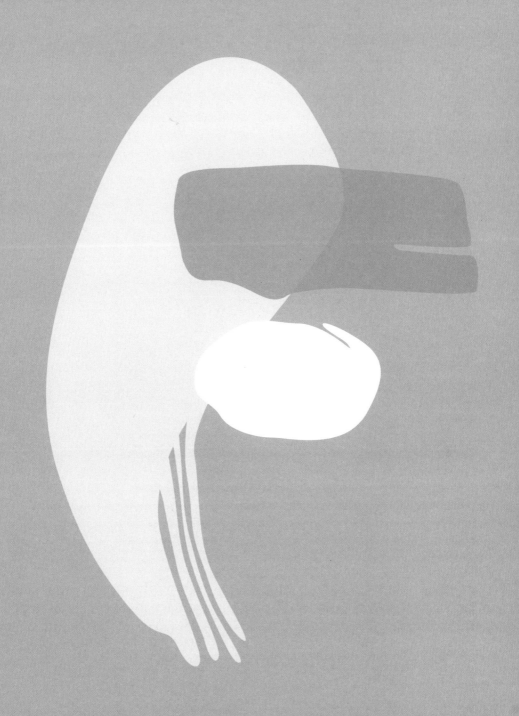

04

Acne

[CHAPTER 11]

Acne is a chronic inflammatory skin condition and it happens to many of us. In fact, about 80–90% of people experience acne in their lifetime,[30] and for many people, well into their 40s. It can impact quality of life, with people reporting low self-esteem, not wanting to leave the house, and even depression or anxiety. What's worse, over half of acne patients think the cause of acne is due to poor hygiene and dirt on their skin.[31] That breaks my heart and I'm certain it contributes to a cycle of harsh treatments and over-cleansing, which in turn makes the breakouts even worse.

It's important to see a dermal clinician, dermatologist or doctor if your acne is moderate to severe, if you're getting scarring, or if it's impacting your mental health. An Australian study[32] found that patients spent an average of AUD$850 on acne management before seeing a dermatologist, and this number was not influenced by income bracket.

What causes acne?

There are four causes of acne:

1. **Individual oil chemistry.** This is the thickness of the oil on your face and how much oil your skin makes. You can have acne without having oily skin.

2. **Blocked or clogged pores.** These are due to build-up of dead skin cells, sweat and oil. At any given time, up to 30% of pores that look clear are clogged, but not all of them turn into acne spots. This is where hormones come in. They influence your oil glands and the way your skin cells shed, which can contribute to build-up.

3. **Acne bacteria (or *Cutibacterium acnes*).** These bacteria exist on all of our skin but only cause trouble for some people.

4. **Inflammation.** This is a complex internal signalling system and is what causes the pain and swelling. An impaired barrier can contribute to inflammation, which is why it's important not to use multiple harsh treatments and to give your skin space to heal.

To treat acne, you need to remove excess oil, unblock the pores, control the acne bacteria and reduce inflammation. This makes it all sound straightforward, but here are a few other things that can help contribute to breakouts:

— stress
— your menstrual cycle
— new skincare or makeup, and hair products
— occlusion from hats and face masks
— touching your face
— infrequent changing of your pillowcase.

Some of these can be controlled, others can't (like my stress levels when writing a book!), but you can always treat with skincare and medicine.

Acne type and severity

Here's a simplified scale you can use to tell how severe your acne is.

NON-INFLAMMATORY	
Closed comedone (whitehead)	Small skin-coloured bumps
Open comedone (blackhead)	Clogged pore with visible dark-coloured plug; this is oxidised sebum
INFLAMMATORY	
Papule	A red bump
Pustule	A red bump with visible pus
Nodule	A large bump, deep in the skin; can be painful. If you get these, you need to see a doctor — they're a high risk for scarring

Mild = Less than 10 inflammatory spots

Moderate = More than 10 inflammatory spots and less than 3 nodules

Severe = More than 10 inflammatory spots and more than 3 nodules

How to treat acne

I've had several recurrences of moderate acne – in my teens, mid-20s, and again very recently. Here's what to look into if you can't see a specialist.

The basics

— **Cleansing.** Do you wear makeup? If so, are you removing it thoroughly? Because it's designed to stay put! Is your cleanser the right one for your skin type? Are you cleansing thoroughly, but gently, twice per day? Try using a cleanser with chemical exfoliants at night, daily to every second day (as tolerated).
— **SPF.** Have you found the right sunscreen for your skin type? (I've reviewed a *lot* and if you search Instagram you can find sunscreen reviews from people with acne-prone skin.) Wearing sunscreen helps prevent the oil on your skin from oxidising and thickening, and it reduces inflammation. It also helps reduce the chances and severity of scarring.
— **Hydration.** Is your skin dehydrated? Are you moisturising your skin morning and night? Try a moisturiser that contains niacinamide – it's gentle and proven to normalise oil production, improve breakouts and the appearance of pores (at 2% concentration).

MY FAVOURITE SUNSCREENS
FOR ACNE-PRONE SKIN

— Biore Aqua Rich Watery Essence SPF 50+ PA++++ (Japan)
— La Roche-Posay Anthelios Invisible SPF 50+ (AU/UK)
— Garnier Advanced Sensitive SPF 50+ (UK/EU)
— Cancer Council Face Day Wear Moisturiser Matte (pink one) SPF 50+ (AU)

Stepping it up

Once you have a basic routine sorted and things are stable for a couple of months, you could try:

— **Adding a chemical exfoliant.** This will help to unclog pores and clear debris to prevent them from clogging again. My favourite chemical exfoliant for breakouts is an AHA/BHA blend. I find they work well together because the AHAs help to normalise the skin's turnover, addressing abnormal cell shedding and making way for the BHA to unclog the pores.

Introduce chemical exfoliants slowly. Use twice per week at first, and then increase as tolerated to every second day – even if the label says to use twice daily. An exfoliant won't work more quickly if you use it more often, it will just overwhelm your skin and you'll be back at square one. Allow three months to see some results. (See Chapter 8 for recommended products.)

— **Adding in more hydration.** You'd be amazed at how much difference a hydrating and healing serum or toner will make in addition to your moisturiser. Especially in winter. It's all about treating the inflammation and hydrating skin in a lightweight way. If you're not already using niacinamide, this could be a way to incorporate it.

What next?

If it's been a while and you're not seeing results or you can't tolerate exfoliants, there are other options.

— **Retinoid (retinol or retinal).** This was a game changer for me, but of course everyone's skin is different. You might initially need to cut back on exfoliation to once per week or less, to prevent sensitivity. Introducing a retinoid requires patience and restraint, but give it 3–6 months and your skin will have transformed.

— **Azelaic acid.** This is another option that's great for breakouts, rosacea and post-inflammatory hyperpigmentation (brown spots after acne). Azelaic acid alone exfoliates your skin but only mildly, so start by using it every second day and work up to daily or even twice daily, at a concentration of 15–20%. It can take 4-plus months to clear up breakouts, so it's not my first choice.

Paula's Choice (US) makes a gentle azelaic acid booster with 10% azelaic acid and some salicylic acid. For a cheaper option, check out the 10% Emulsion from Naturium or the Azelaic Acid Suspension 10% from The Ordinary.

Here are other at-home treatments you can try:

— **Clay masks.** They're designed to pull excess oil out of your pores and bring existing blemishes to a head, and can sometimes contain exfoliating acids or acne-targeting ingredients like sulphur. I like to use clay masks if I haven't done my skincare the night before or after strenuous activity.
— **LED masks.** These were developed by NASA to help astronauts' bodies recover from the distress of space. For acne, both blue and red light are helpful. Blue light kills acne bacteria and red light soothes, speeds up repair and builds collagen, which can help prevent scarring. At-home LED masks are expensive, however, so at this point it's probably worth going to the doctor instead.

MY FAVOURITE CLAY MASKS

— NIOD Flavanone Mud (Global): Wonderful for treating dullness, drawing out any brewing spots and shrinking existing spots. Be warned: there's quite a tingle.
— Mecca Max X-Zit Strategy (AU): Inexpensive and works quickly to shrink spots
— Dr Dennis Gross Blemish Solutions Clarifying Mask (Global): Calms and heals as it draws out excess oil

How to spot treat

Spot treating is great for speeding up the clearance of an existing spot, but it won't help prevent more spots. It's also very tempting to do too much and make it worse. Don't pick at spots or try to pop them. It never helps, unless it's done by a professional and there is a higher risk of scarring. There are several options for spot treating:

— **Pimple patches.** If you're prone to picking, pimple patches are perfect for you. A pimple patch is a hydrocolloid bandage designed specifically to treat pimples. Hydrocolloid is used in wound healing and draws out fluid from the wound while protecting it from the environment. In this instance, the environment includes *you*. Pimple patches are best for treating papules or pustules and they come with or without acne-targeted ingredients.
— **Clay and sulphur masks.** These help draw spots out.
— **Benzoyl peroxide.** This is another well-researched spot treatment but always go for the lowest concentration possible – 2.5%, not 10%. Higher concentrations don't work any better in most cases and they're more irritating. And we need our skin to *not* be irritated, because we need it to repair a wound.

MY FAVOURITE SPOT TREATMENT

LED, blue and red, is my absolute favourite spot treatment for any inflamed acne. It shortens a spot's life from a week to a few days, and a nodule that would normally last a month for me will clear in a week or two.

The Dr Dennis Gross SpotLite Acne Treatment Device with blue and red LED technology is one of the more affordable options available.

On that note, no scrubs please! Breakouts don't happen because your skin isn't clean. It's a medical condition. Using something abrasive on a wound will irritate it, potentially spread the infection and make things worse. Wounds heal best when they're kept moisturised.

How to treat acne scarring

Let's first get the terminology right, because there are different types of acne scarring, with different treatment options. There's no point in treating indented scarring without getting the breakouts themselves under control, because you'll just end up with more scarring to treat.

Flat scars

Flat scars fall into two categories: PIE and PIH.

PIE is post-inflammatory erythema, which are the red or purple marks left behind after a spot – like a red mark you might have after a cut has healed. They happen due to inflammatory changes to blood vessels in the area while the spot was active.

You can help these marks fade more quickly at home by using sunscreen with retinoids, azelaic acid or niacinamide, and barrier-repairing, antioxidant ingredients. In-clinic options such as peels or lasers also help speed up the process.

PIH is post-inflammatory hyperpigmentation, which are brown marks left behind after a spot, more likely seen in medium to deep skin tones. You can experience both PIH and PIE at once, but PIH occurs in skin types that overproduce melanin when inflamed. You must use sunscreen to treat these and azelaic acid is helpful for both acne and pigmented scarring. Because this is hyperpigmentation, look for brightening ingredients. Again, you can speed up treatment in-clinic with peels or lasers. Ask your treating clinician what's best for you.

Indented scars

Indented scars happen when inflammation from the spot degrades collagen in your skin's dermis.

Most indented scars are ice pick scars – they're v-shaped, narrow and go quite deep, sometimes as far as the hypodermis. You can also get boxcar scars, which are wider and round or oval-shaped. Then there are rolling scars, which are the widest (up to 5 mm) and give skin a ripply texture.

Indented scars aren't super treatable at home but sunscreen will help preserve your collagen and retinoids can help remodel it. There are also many in-clinic options. Ask your treating doctor or dermal clinician. This is the kind of thing you need to go to a medical clinic for.

Key takeaways

— Acne is an inflammatory condition of your skin. It's a medical condition, not caused by poor hygiene or diet.

— All acne is influenced by hormones and is a result of four factors: individual oil chemistry, clogged pores, acne bacteria and inflammation.

— Spot treating is great for speeding up the clearance of an existing spot, but it won't help prevent more spots.

— Don't use scrubs to treat breakouts. Using something abrasive on a wound will irritate it, potentially spread the infection and make things worse. Wounds heal best when they're kept moisturised.

— There are many options you can try at home to treat breakouts and acne, but if it's severe please see a doctor, to reduce the risk of scarring.

Wrinkles and retinoids

[CHAPTER 12]

It's one thing to acknowledge the inevitability of getting older and another thing entirely to accept it and be positive about it when it's happening to your own face. Our culture is obsessed with youth, especially in women, and the self-loathing we learn as we grow up runs deep. They get us young. For that reason, I want you to really think about your language when you talk about age-related changes to your and others' skin. I'm not perfect. I'm trying to unlearn it too. What I never want to hear again is a statement like 'you shouldn't sunbake because you will be ugly and wrinkly'.

You're going to get wrinkles someday. Don't do your future self a disservice by speaking about them in this way. Can we discuss the physiology of skin wrinkling and how to minimise it without going down the patriarchal road of self-loathing? Maybe not. Maybe the two concepts are inextricably linked. I'm going to do my best.

In this chapter we're going to talk about what's changed in the skin to create these conditions so that we can understand how to best optimise our skin's health.

Our culture is obsessed with youth, especially in women, and the self-loathing we learn as we grow up runs deep.

Why do we get wrinkles?

It's quite simple. Your face and body make the same movements all the time and as our biological functions slow down and we accumulate more sun exposure, oxidative stress and glycation, the quality of our skin's collagen and elastin proteins will degrade.

—

Collagen is the structural protein that gives skin a smooth texture and elastin is what helps it snap back.

The degradation of collagen and elastin means that skin can't bounce back as easily from loss of support and elasticity. So the expressions we make start to etch lines into our skin. If you smile with your eyes, you might see lines forming in that area. Gorgeous. Or if your eyesight isn't the best you might squint a lot and start to see a line forming between your brows.

As we lose collagen and elastin over time, the dermis thins and cannot support the epidermis as well as before. That's when we see wrinkles, in areas not involved in expression.

There are plenty of opportunities to support your skin and give it the nutrients it needs to keep making that all-important collagen and elastin. But remember: your life is a long journey to loving yourself.

WRINKLES AND RETINOIDS

Strategies for protecting and smoothing skin

— **Protect your skin from further environmental stress.**
Now that you understand the cause of the lines, you'll be better equipped to properly preserve your skin. This means committing to sunscreen to protect from UV. It means using antioxidants to protect from the effects of other visible light, pollution, oxidative stress and glycation. It also means eating antioxidants too. Doing this will give you great results. That's because your skin now has spare energy to heal and rebuild because it isn't as inflamed and using all its energy to repair the ongoing damage.
— **Hydrate.** We often see fine lines when our skin is dehydrated. Simply giving it the water it needs will plump out those fine lines.
— **Reverse the damage.** The best-studied ingredients that reverse damage are retinoids. Others proven to help with symptoms of photo-ageing are vitamin C, vitamin B3 (niacinamide) and AHAs. Lesser-studied but helpful ingredients include DNA repair enzymes, green tea, caffeine and resveratrol. If you're already using these, you could also try peptides and growth factors. Peptides can be helpful for elasticity and are well tolerated compared to strong retinoids.

Retinoids

'Retinoid' is an umbrella term for compounds related to vitamin A. If you're after skincare that will reverse damage, retinoids are the gold standard. Here are some proven effects of vitamin A:

— stimulates collagen production
— promotes a thicker dermis and more organised epidermis
— helps prevent and reverse UV-associated changes to blood vessels
— helps prevent collagen and elastin breakdown
— helps normalise cell turnover, reducing clogged pores and treating acne
— signals skin to better hydrate itself by stimulating hyaluronic acid production
— promotes great antioxidant activity
— shrinks oil glands (oral isotretinoin)
— helps with hyperpigmentation (especially prescription tretinoin and retinal)
— improves fine and deep wrinkles
— some have an antibacterial effect (retinaldehyde).

Forms of vitamin A

In your diet, vitamin A is found in meat, eggs and dairy. A lot of the vitamin A you eat also comes from a provitamin A called beta-carotene (in carrots, tomato, broccoli and spinach). It's good for your eyesight as well as your skin.

In skincare, vitamin A comes in a few forms:

— retinyl acetate
— retinyl palmitate
— hydroxypinacolone retinoate
— retinyl propionate

- retinyl retinoate (two clinical trials compared 0.06% retinyl retinoate to 0.75% retinol and found it gave better results)
- retinol (how our skin naturally stores its vitamin A; effective at as little as 0.01%, with 1% being the most you'll find)
- retinaldehyde/retinal (available at 0.01%–0.2%; meant to work eleven times faster than retinol).

In your skin, some vitamin A is stored as beta-carotene, some as retinol and some as retinyl acetate. In order for these to influence your cells, they are converted to retinoic acid.

The forms below are prescription strength and should be discussed with your prescribing doctor.

- retinoic acid/tretinoin
- adapalene, tazorac
- oral isotretinoin (Roaccutane/Accutane).

RETINOIDS	
Over the counter (weakest to strongest, least to most irritating)	Retinyl Acetate
	Hydroxypinacolone Retinoate
	Retinyl Palmitate
	Retinyl Propionate
	Retinyl Retinoate
	Retinol
	Retinaldehyde/Retinal
Prescription (more irritating)	Retinoic Acid (Tretinoin)
	Adapalene (Differin)
	Tazorac
	Isotretinoin (Oral - Accutane/ Roaccutane)

How to introduce retinoids

Too much vitamin A applied to the skin can be irritating. If you go too strong or too fast, your skin might freak out, break out, become overly sensitive or compromised, flake and/or feel irritated. I don't want you to buy something and end up unable to use it. Irritation from retinoids can take 24–48 hours to show up due to the specific inflammatory pathways that excess retinoids trigger in skin.

Start by incorporating a measured (pea size) amount once per week, to learn how it affects *your* skin. When I first started retinoids, I used it once per week for three months. After six months the texture of my skin had transformed and I stopped breaking out completely. It's a long game, especially if you're acne-prone, or have sensitive skin or rosacea.

Over time, your skin will build a tolerance. This doesn't mean you need more to have the same effects; on the contrary, it means you'll get quicker results from the same amount and can therefore up your dosage to get even more benefits.

Can you tell I'm a huge fan?

There's no 'right age' to start retinoids. You might notice larger pores, fine lines forming and less hydration around your mid-20s, so this might be a good time to start. But if you're experiencing clogged pores and breakouts, retinoids can help at any age.

ROUTINE: RETINOIDS

This is a guide for use of 0.5% retinol and up. Gentler products can be introduced more quickly as tolerated. If you're using a prescription retinoid, follow the advice of your doctor.

Retinoid days (once per week for at least a month, work up to 2+ × per week)

AM

1. Cleanse (optional)
2. Antioxidant serum
3. SPF

PM

1. Double cleanse
2. Eye cream
3. Hydrating serum, moisturiser
4. Retinoid (pea size – one pump)
5. Healing balm

Non-retinoid days

AM

1. Cleanse (optional)
2. Antioxidant serum
3. SPF

PM

1. Double cleanse
2. Eye cream
3. Hydrating serum, moisturiser
4. Healing balm (optional)

There are no exfoliating acids or other skin-challenging active ingredients because we're taking the most delicate approach possible. Retinoids perform many functions so you don't really need other actives.

Which retinoid ingredient should you choose?

Here's a shortcut to choosing retinoid ingredients.

IF YOU'RE ...	TRY ...
Extremely sensitive, or after low-key smoothing or something very gentle where you won't notice any side effects	Retinyl propionate or retinyl retinoate – these derivatives are proven to have some effects with less irritation
Ready for a slight challenge and want fabulous results	Retinol or retinaldehyde – start at once per week
After more, or suffering from severe acne or sun damage	Chatting to a doctor – you might be a candidate for prescription retinoids
Pregnant or breastfeeding	Over-the-counter retinoids – current evidence suggests that people who are pregnant or breastfeeding should avoid prescription retinoids, but over-the-counter products are OK[33]

And no plant oils or extracts! They won't give you enough vitamin A in the doses you'll need.

What concentration should you look for?

Not all products will disclose the concentration, but here's a guide to how much you'll need in order to see an effect.

INGREDIENT	CONCENTRATION
Retinyl propionate	At least 0.3%
Retinyl retinoate	At least 0.05%
Retinol	From 0.1% to 1%
Retinal	From 0.01% to 0.2%

MY FAVOURITE RETINOID PRODUCTS

— Olay's Regenerist Retinol 24 Night Moisturiser, Night Serum and Eye Cream
— Verso Night Cream
— Medik8 r-Retinoate Day & Night Youth-Activating Cream
— SkinCeuticals Retinol 0.3%, 0.5% and 1.0%
— Paula's Choice 1% Retinol Booster
— Paula's Choice RESIST 0.1% Intensive Wrinkle-Repair Serum
— La Roche-Posay Retinol B3 Serum
— First Aid Beauty Skin Lab Retinol Serum
— Medik8 Crystal Retinal 6
— Avène A-Oxitive Night Peeling Cream
— Osmosis Clarify Blemish Retinal Serum
— Allies of Skin Retinal & Peptides Repair Night Cream

How long until you see results?

My advice? Take pictures. It might take four weeks or less to see improvements, three months for people to start noticing (but if they're rude enough to comment on your appearance, send them my way), and six months to a year for major changes. It's not a race!

Eye cream

Common issues around the eye area include fine lines and wrinkles, loss of elasticity in the eyelid, dark circles, dehydrated/dry skin and puffiness or 'bags'. These changes happen due largely to the sun so make sure to wear sunglasses and sunscreen.

If your skin is dry or dehydrated, use a moisturiser or sunscreen. If you want to tighten the eyelid, you'll need to improve the skin's elasticity. Look for something hydrating with retinoid and/or peptides. If your eye area gets puffy, don't use a thick cream at night. This can make it worse. Try a serum instead. I've also found caffeine to be a really helpful ingredient for quick de-puffing.

If you have visible dark circles, treatment will depend on the cause. Dark circles can appear as a result of hyperpigmentation (brown discolouration), which is best treated with brightening ingredients such as niacinamide or vitamin C. Dark circles may be vascular from muscle and blood vessels showing through the thin under-eye skin (purple discolouration), which can be treated with retinoids to thicken the skin, and caffeine to constrict the vessels. Dark circles can also be structural from the shape and placement of bone, fat and muscle around the eye. There's not much to be done about a structural dark circle apart from surgery. You might experience more than one of these – or all three like me. (Realistically, my favourite treatment for dark circles is concealer.)

Key takeaways

— Wrinkles happen when our skin loses elasticity over time, due largely to the sun. The best treatment is prevention so make sure you're applying that sunscreen daily.

— Retinoids (aka vitamin A) are amazing for a number of skin concerns, but introduce them carefully as they can be irritating for the skin. It's a long game — it can take up to six months to see major changes.

— When choosing an eye cream, think about your skin concerns. Are you targeting fine lines and wrinkles, loss of elasticity, dark circles, dehydrated skin, puffiness, or all of the above?

Hyperpigmentation

[CHAPTER 13]

The colour of your skin is a mix of brown pigment (melanin), red and blue from blood, and yellow from your diet. People with dark and light skin have the same amount of melanocytes (melanin-producing cells), only in light skin they're less active and produce less melanin. Melanin has a protective role for skin, which is why darker skin has a lower risk of skin cancer, but hyperpigmentation is more likely.

What is hyperpigmentation?

Hyperpigmentation occurs when your skin produces too much melanin in an uneven way. Both keratinocytes and melanocytes pick up melanin and store it around the cell's nucleus (where the DNA is) as a 'cap' to protect the DNA from UV damage. Leftover melanin gets 'dropped' and accumulates in the space between cells.

This can appear as a dark spot or patch after a blemish, friction or wound (hyperpigmentation from inflammation), as melasma (hyperpigmentation from hormones, usually in a symmetrical pattern), or as freckles, sunspots or even cancer (hyperpigmentation from sun damage). It can end up as deep in the skin as the dermis, where it's harder to treat.

It's important to have regular skin checks with a GP or dermatologist because hyperpigmentation can sometimes be a sign of developing cancer. Removing hyperpigmentation will eliminate the visible signs without removing the cancer, which can develop unchecked. For this reason, it's important to go to a clinic that has a dermatologist and dermal clinician on-site. Your clinician should ask about your last skin check before any in-clinic depigmenting treatments.

How to treat hyperpigmentation

The first thing to do in treating hyperpigmentation is to eliminate the cause as much as you can. Treat acne or any other contributing inflammatory condition, balance hormones where you can (you'll need to see a doctor if this applies to you) and protect yourself from the sun. Some products and ingredients treat both acne and associated post-inflammatory hyperpigmentation.

After treating any underlying causes, the strategy for hyperpigmentation is to interrupt the melanin's production or its transfer from the melanocytes to the keratinocytes, and to encourage faster cell turnover in order to remove the pigmented cells and replace them with new ones.

You don't want to create sensitivity in your skin, particularly with skin prone to post-inflammatory hyperpigmentation, because inflammation = pigmentation. Be mindful of ingredients that are less kind to your skin and seek clinical guidance if you think you need prescription products.

Don't push your skin too far and be patient. It's a challenging skincare goal. Take it one day at a time.

Effective ingredients for hyperpigmentation

When treating hyperpigmentation with over-the-counter skincare, I find that products with a mix of ingredients are best (rather than one-hit-wonder-type products). Here are some ingredients that help hyperpigmentation by limiting production and transfer of pigment:

— niacinamide
— hydroquinone (gold standard, not to be used more than three months at a time)
— N-acetyl glucosamine
— arbutin
— hexylresorcinol
— potassium azeloyl diglycinate
— azelaic acid (good for melasma and PIH, not so good for sunspots)
— green tea
— vitamin C
— diglucosyl gallic acid
— tranexamic acid
— kojic acid
— licorice root
— viniferine
— ellagic acid
— 4-n-butylresorcinol
— resveratrol
— acetyl glycyl beta-alanine.

The following ingredients will encourage cell turnover (you might already be using these in your exfoliant step):

retinoids:
— retinol
— retinal
— prescription

acids:
— lactic
— glycolic
— salicylic
— tartaric
— malic
— mandelic
— PHAs

MY FAVOURITE PIGMENTATION PRODUCTS

— NIOD RE: Pigment
— Sachi Triphala Pigmentation Corrector
— La Clinica Intensive Correction Serum Level 2
— Caudalie Vinoperfect Radiance Serum

How long does it take to treat pigmentation?

Expect to see a difference anywhere between four weeks and three months. After three months, if the improvement isn't noticeable or fast enough, there are in-clinic treatments available to speed up treatment, like lasers or peels.

ROUTINE: PIGMENTATION

AM

1. Cleanse (optional)
2. Antioxidant serum
3. SPF

PM

1. Cleanse
2. Second cleanse with acids (if tolerated)
3. Pigment serum
4. Moisturiser/Healing balm

Weekly

— 2–3 × retinoids
— 2–3 × acids (if you aren't acid cleansing)

In-clinic treatments

In-clinic hyperpigmentation treatments include peels, lasers and IPL (intense pulsed light). Your clinician should organise a treatment plan that incorporates both skincare and procedures. It's also important to have a doctor perform a skin cancer check beforehand.

When undergoing in-clinic treatments, make sure to continue doing at-home treatments. If you're not using skincare daily to block hyperpigmentation, you won't get the full benefits of your clinical treatments (and they're not cheap).

Key takeaways

— The biggest contributor to unwanted dark spots and uneven skin tone is the sun. Hyperpigmentation will improve just by committing to sunscreen.

— It's important not to push your skin too far as stressed skin can create excess pigment too.

— Clinical guidance from your dermatologist, dermal clinician or aesthetician is very helpful. They have a solid understanding of which treatments will work best for your skin.

Skincare mistakes

[CHAPTER 14]

Skincare mistakes? We're all guilty of them. But it doesn't mean we have to keep making them. Here are some mistakes you might be unintentionally making with respect to your skincare and some tips on how to fix them.

Not using your sunscreen right

Do ...

— use other methods of protection – hats, sunglasses, clothing, staying in the shade.
— use enough sunscreen. That's a ¼ teaspoon for your face; ½ teaspoon for neck and ears; or 1 teaspoon for your whole head if you have no hair. Apply 1 teaspoon per limb, 1 teaspoon for your trunk at the front and 1 teaspoon for your back. Think about these amounts if you're using a spray sunscreen – how will you know you're wearing enough? Make sure to apply a couple of layers.

— reapply every two hours or after swimming or sweating. The film that your sunscreen forms is broken up by sweat and oil on your skin.

Do not …

— spend too long in the sun. Sunscreen does not make you invincible. If your job involves entire days in the sun, that's an OHS issue and you need to wear protective clothing.
— mix your sunscreen with another product. Don't mix sunscreen with foundation to make tinted sunscreen, don't mix sunscreen with highlight for glow, don't mix sunscreen with liquid bronzer. Sunscreen must form an even film on your skin and diluting it can destabilise that film, leading to patchy protection.
— rely on the SPF in your foundation. You need a ¼ teaspoon of sunscreen on your face, or close to. No one wears that much foundation (if you do, I guess you're exempt). Measure it out if you feel brave.
— use powder SPF for touch-ups. How are you going to get a ¼ teaspoon of that on your face? It's not enough protection.
— forget about your neck and chest. These areas get exposed to the sun too!

Product pilling

Has this ever happened to you? You're applying your layers of skincare and suddenly it starts pilling and rolling off in little balls. Now you have to take it all off and start from scratch. What happened?

The cause is usually using too many different products, applying too much of each product, not letting layers dry or too much rubbing. Sometimes it's product incompatibility, and occasionally it's just a terrible product. When I review sunscreens, I intentionally rub them in for longer, to test if they ball up. Silicones and silica are sometimes the culprit because they form a film. If you keep rubbing in while the film is forming, it can lift off and take everything else with it.

Try the following to reduce the chances of your skincare pilling:

— Apply serums to damp skin, to help them absorb better.
— Apply thinnest to thickest.
— Don't apply too much of each product.
— Minimise the number of products in your routine.
— Let your layers dry in between.
— Don't rub too much.
— Know that face oils can interfere with the films formed by silicones. That's why oil cleansers demolish makeup so easily. Try adding your face oil to your moisturiser, instead of layering it.

Sometimes if you mist (with water or your favourite skincare mist) over the top and pat it all back in, you can avoid having to remove all your layers and starting again – unless it's sunscreen. You always need to apply enough sunscreen.

Exfoliating skin when it's flaky

When your skin looks dry and starts flaking, it can be tempting to scrub it off. But let's examine what's really going on here. The cells along the top layer of your skin aren't sitting in their usual uniform layers. They're lifting off and this means your barrier might not be as airtight as it can be. Exfoliating further can exacerbate the problem (eczema is inflammation from a chronically impaired barrier). Try hydrating your skin instead. Add a hydrating serum under your moisturiser or a couple drops of face oil on top.

Incompatible ingredients

Maybe you aren't sure if you can use your exfoliating serum with a certain peptide. Or you're worried about clashing actives in your products. So how do you know if the ingredients in your skincare routine are compatible?

If you want to do two things but both steps are 'takers', you might want to reconsider doing both. For example, I wouldn't use an acid exfoliant and retinoids on the same night. If your skin is used to strong ingredients and you're sure combining them won't cause unnecessary irritation, then go ahead (within reason, of course).

If you want the benefits of a couple of different ingredient categories, try to find a two-in-one product instead of combining products. This way, all of the ingredients have been formulated to work together optimally and you don't end up with a 25-step routine you can't remember (been there).

—

Ask yourself: Am I giving back to my skin or taking from it with this step?

Acne treatment

Harsh cleansing, over-cleansing and scrubbing

An acne lesion is an inflamed, clogged pore. A wound. Would you scrub an inflamed cut? No. I think this behaviour stems from the assumption that acne means your skin is dirty. That's completely false. Stripping your skin with scrubs and harsh cleansers is one of the worst things you can do, and acne will only get worse if you over-scrub and over-wash. If someone tells you that you need to 'wash your face', they don't belong in your life. Who asked for their advice, anyway?

'Get some sun'

Heard this one before? It's wrong. All the sun will do is contribute to inflammation, slow healing time and worsen the dark spots that are left behind after a blemish.

Emulating someone else's skincare routine

You've done the exploratory quiz and figured out your skin needs and skin goals, so you know there are a lot of factors to account for in your own skin. I'm all for sharing product recommendations, but we all have different needs, preferences, temperaments and lifestyles. Not to mention bodies.

I have freckles, underlying sun damage and very sensitive skin. I have experienced acne, perioral dermatitis, and now rosacea too. My skin is otherwise pretty typical – it can be oily on the nose, forehead and chin; it can be dehydrated and dry on the neck and cheeks. I'm not prone to wrinkles (yet), but I'm seeing loss of elasticity and texture from old acne scarring at the jawline and sides of my mouth, as well as in my eyelids. Especially on the driver's side. And I love experimenting on my face with in-clinic treatments.

Everyone has a story for their skin. Someone might recommend a product that worked for their acne but won't think to mention all of the other factors. The rest of their routine could be really nourishing and help them to tolerate a product that's otherwise quite harsh. Get to know your skin and how to meet its needs instead of emulating someone else's skincare routine entirely.

Key takeaways

— Be sun-smart and apply sunscreen liberally. Your skin will thank you in years to come.

— If you want the benefits of a couple of different ingredient categories, try to find a two-in-one product instead of combining products.

— Make sure your skincare routine is about your wants and needs, not someone else's. Question everything.

Seeing a professional

Let me take you back to the Australian dermatology clinic study that found that new patients spent an average of AUD$850 on acne management in the six months before seeing a dermatologist (with this number not influenced by income bracket). It concluded that treating acne has a financial impact on patients and seeing a dermatologist earlier could save money.

But it's not just money. Many of us don't know where to start or what to expect when seeing a professional for skin-related issues.

In Australia, there are beauty therapists, dermal clinicians, dermatology nurses, GPs, dermatologists and telehealth doctors. In the US and UK, there are also aestheticians and telehealth services for skin. There are also people who work in retail selling skincare and customer service reps for online retailers, who can help you choose products. At every level, people have varying levels of experience and knowledge.

FAQs

When should I see a professional?

It depends. You might have your basic skincare routine down, you've added in a treatment step here and there, but you're not sure if you're getting it right. Or maybe it's been a few months and you're not seeing any results. The next step could be to see an expert.

See a doctor ASAP if you have a skin condition and it's impacting your quality of life. I'm not sure who brainwashed everyone into thinking skin and mental health are less serious than any other ailment, but I'd like a word with them and it won't be polite.

What can a GP do?

A GP can diagnose acne, perioral dermatitis, rosacea and other skin conditions, and provide treatment and advice, or a referral to a dermatologist if required. They can also prescribe medications such as creams, hormonal treatments and antibiotics for acne. (In Australia, a GP can't prescribe isotretinoin for acne. You'll need to see a dermatologist for this because it must be monitored by a skin expert.) GPs can also conduct skin checks so make sure to book in for a yearly skin check.

Your experience can vary greatly between doctors. All doctors are qualified to understand risks and manage complications, but a medical degree doesn't cover skin to a great extent, which is why many take on postgraduate study. Any doctor in Australia can call themselves a cosmetic doctor or even cosmetic surgeon, so always enquire about credentials and experience. Dermatologists have specific mandates and years of training.

What does a beauty therapist or dermal therapist do?

In Australia, a beauty therapist can have qualifications that have taken months up to a year to complete. This is the equivalent to an aesthetician in the US or UK. You can go to a beauty therapist for treatments, LED and an objective opinion on your skin's progress.

What does a dermal clinician do?

A dermal clinician has studied a four-year Bachelor of Health Science degree with practical components and is a more formalised version of a medical aesthetician. Unlike a doctor or nurse, dermal clinicians don't have to be registered with AHPRA (Australian Health Practitioner Regulation Agency) and are not bound by its guidelines; however, this is something the Australian Society of Dermal Clinicians is pushing to change.

Dermal clinicians can provide medical facial treatments (e.g. laser for rosacea or peels for acne scarring) and cosmetic treatments (e.g. laser or microneedling for rejuvenation). They can help you choose the right products to treat skin conditions such as acne, rosacea, psoriasis, eczema and dermatitis, but they can't prescribe retinoids or other prescription creams such as antibiotics.

What does a dermatologist do?

Dermatologists are doctors that have undertaken a further five years of postgraduate study to qualify as medical specialists in skin. They're the experts!

A dermatologist can help manage the treatment of skin, hair and nails. They can assist with difficult, recurring skin conditions and are more experienced in identifying what's going on with your skin and recognising health issues. A dermatologist can also help with hair loss. They can run blood tests to check for any deficiencies that might be related to your concerns.

What about telehealth skin services?

Telehealth skin services are pretty cool and I wish they were around when I was growing up. You can either send photos or have a video call with your doctor, and they prescribe a custom product for your skin concerns that's shipped to your home. In Australia, there's Skin.Software and The Secret, in the UK there's Dermatica and Skin+me, and in the US there's Curology.

Who do I see for a facial?

First think about what you want. Are you after a gentle facial? Maybe a mask and some extractions (which involves medically squeezing out your pores)? Or perhaps a discussion about what you could add to or change about your skincare? Then a skin clinic with beauty therapists might be what you're after.

If you're after something relaxing but more results-driven — such as a peel, needling or a laser — visit a clinic with beauty therapists and dermal clinicians.

If you're after more medical results, find a clinic with a dermatologist on site. I've found that to be a good shortcut to getting a dermatologist appointment. If your concern calls for a dermatologist, they'll book you in with theirs as an existing patient following a cosmetic consult.

Safety

How can you tell if a provider is qualified to perform a particular treatment safely and effectively? Aside from enquiring about qualifications, it's helpful to ask the practitioner what their plan is if something were to go wrong. In the case that something does go wrong, you'll want access to medical treatment.

The Australian Society of Dermal Clinicians website has an excellent list of questions to ask your treatment provider before moving forward with a treatment plan. Head to https://www.dermalclinicians.com.au/questions-to-ask

See a doctor ASAP if you have a skin condition and it's impacting your quality of life.

SEEING A PROFESSIONAL

Key takeaways

— When choosing a skin professional, think about what you want to achieve and who might have the best qualifications to get you there.

— See a doctor ASAP if you have a skin condition and it's impacting your quality of life. Be aware that your experience may vary greatly between doctors.

— When looking into skin treatments, if the price is too good to be true, it probably is.

The other stuff

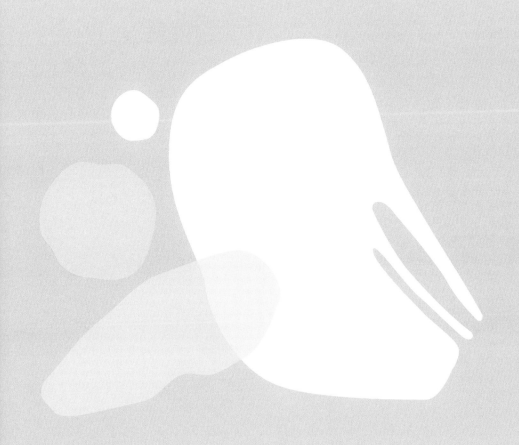

05

Skin and diet

[CHAPTER 16]

Content warning: This chapter contains discussion around eating disorders and body dysmorphia. If you are experiencing digestive symptoms, suspected food intolerance or allergies, talk to your GP or a registered dietician. If you are experiencing body dysmorphia or an eating disorder, talk to your GP, psychologist or psychiatrist, or contact one of the organisations below.

Australia
— Butterfly Foundation: 1800 33 4673
— Lifeline: 13 11 14
— National Eating Disorders Collaboration:
  https://nedc.com.au/

UK
— Beat Eating Disorders: 0808 801 0677
— National Suicide Helpline: UK 0800 689 5652

US
— National Eating Disorders Association: 800 931-2237
— National Suicide Prevention Hotline: 1 800 273 8255

We've all seen it. A celebrity or influencer insisting that going gluten-free and vegan cured their breakouts, rosacea, eczema, tax debt and relationship problems. Never mind their on-call dermatologist or professional-grade LED bed at home. But we trust their claims because we're socialised to trust and value good-looking people. Sigh.

This kind of unsolicited, ill-informed diet advice is harmful. Diet culture has a vicious grip on our society, and by diet culture I mean the way that we, as a society, value staying thin ahead of our physical and emotional health. Body dysmorphia can and does lead to disordered eating, and when your skin isn't where you'd like it to be, feelings of sadness and anxiety can arise. Critically examining your skin is no different to critically examining your body. It's not a good place to be.

We know that getting essential nutrients is great for your skin. By the same token, arbitrarily cutting out an entire food group because a celeb said they quit gluten fails to consider your own body's needs.

—

There's no scientific consensus that changing what you eat will treat acne.

So we're not going to talk about cutting any food groups out. If you suspect that some foods may be linked to a skin condition, or if your skin is impacting your emotional health and self-esteem, please see your GP. They can refer you to a registered dietitian, dermatologist and/or psychologist.

What we are going to talk about are the nutrients that are great for skin. I've experienced some difficult times when it comes to what I eat and my relationship with my body, and coming out on the other side, my strategy is always to add foods rather than limit them.

Nutrients that are helpful for your skin

Omega-3s

Omega-3s help with skin, heart health and brain function. Unfortunately our bodies can't make omega-3 fatty acids (alpha-linolenic acid/ALA, eicosapentaenoic acid/EPA and docosahexaenoic acid/DHA), so add them into your diet by having three servings of oily fish per week, such as tuna or salmon. Alternatively, try flaxseed, hempseeds, chia seeds, walnuts, or take fish oil supplements. Vegans can add omega-3s through flaxseed oil or omega-3 supplements made from algae.

Dietary fibre

Get your dietary fibre through having five servings of fruit and vegetables per day. Fibre is also found in beans (legumes), oats, brown rice, high-fibre bread and pasta. I sneak a couple of servings of vegetables into my breakfast smoothie for a head start. Fibre keeps your digestive tract healthy.

Antioxidants

Yes! Eating antioxidants helps your skin. Some even help your skin resist sun damage (in addition to, not instead of, sunscreen and sun-safe behaviour), such as tomatoes, berries, watermelon and pomegranate.

When you decide a food is 'bad', you tend to think of yourself as 'bad' if you eat it. Food keeps you alive – it has no moral value.

Nutrition and acne

There are many factors to consider in the treatment of acne before turning to diet. So why are we told to cut out sugar and dairy in order to treat acne?

In a nutshell, high GI foods and dairy can *indirectly* contribute to oil production and abnormal shedding of dead skin cells in your pores,[34] so there's more oil and dead cells to remove, otherwise the pore will clog. Probiotics and omega-3 fatty acids do help, as can targeted skincare, which means you can step away from the unnecessarily restrictive dietary advice.

Dr Dennis Gross has said that if his patients insist they changed something about how they eat and it's helping with their acne, he'll leave them to it – even if there isn't supporting evidence. At the end of the day, do what works for you.

Nutrition and rosacea

Some people find that their rosacea is triggered by certain foods and drinks, such as spicy foods or alcohol. Unlike acne, however, the effect is documented and more immediate. This can happen if your rosacea is sensitive to heat (from hot drinks or spicy food), if your blood vessels are dilated (alcohol dilates blood vessels), or if food contains a lot of histamine (e.g. tomato, eggplant, spinach, alcoholic drinks such as wine, or fermented foods such as sauerkraut, kimchi, yoghurt and cheese), which can also dilate blood vessels and is involved in inflammation.

Everyone is different, so seek advice from your GP, dermatologist or dietitian.

To supplement or not to supplement?

Supplements don't have the same burden of evidence as medicines. They don't have to be as well studied, because the implications of taking them are less serious. This is generally fine, but did you know that supplements can cause drug reactions? Always tell your doctor what supplements you are currently taking along with your medications.

It's important to remember that *the dose makes the poison*. Take vitamin A as an example. It's a fat-soluble vitamin, meaning your body can store it (unlike vitamins B and C). If you're vitamin A deficient (which is rare), your vision and fertility may be impacted, but too much can cause joint pain and even birth defects. Rest assured, there is a very large window – the recommended intake is 700 mcg per day (which most people get from their diets) and the upper safe limit is 3000 mcg per day, more than four times that.

Many skin, hair and nail supplements contain biotin, or vitamin B7. Deficiency is uncommon but it can cause hair loss; however, taking biotin won't help your hair unless you're actually deficient. It's better to see a doctor, have a blood test, and treat the actual cause of hair loss. High levels of biotin from supplements can cause breakouts and interfere with blood tests for other conditions, including for thyroid and heart function. Please don't take it without advice from a doctor.

Collagen supplements are low-risk and there's some evidence showing that they help with skin hydration and collagen quality, at 3–10 g per day.[35] They've been widely used in Japan for a long time – you can find it there in collagen drinks and gummies.

There's also a tendency in Western media to discount traditional medicines such as Ayurveda or traditional Chinese medicine, perhaps due to the 'lack of evidence' (that is, evidence in English) or their appropriation by advocates of new-age woo woo. I'm pro-evidence, but research is expensive and pharmaceutical companies are usually the ones who pay for it because they've patented the experimental compound and hope to recoup the R&D investment. You can't really patent a traditional herb that's been used for thousands of years. A lack of evidence doesn't necessarily mean it doesn't work, only that it hasn't been proven.

Key takeaways

— Your skin's function is largely independent of what you eat. There's no evidence that changing what you eat or following a restrictive meal plan will treat acne.

— If you do want to target what you eat, try incorporating more omega-3 fatty acids and dietary fibre into your diet.

— Supplements are optional. Always check with your doctor first.

Body care

[CHAPTER 17]

So far, we've talked a lot about making sure your face is happy and well looked after, but what about your body? There's skin there too.

The skin on your body is 2–3 times thicker than the face and it turns over more slowly, so you can afford to be more aggressive with it. Jagged acne scrubs you couldn't use on your face because they were too rough? Great for the body. A cleanser that was too harsh? Makes for an excellent body wash. Acid toners that destroyed your face? Again, perfect for the body. It's a great way to use products that would otherwise go in the bin. Unless you have eczema, in which case be as gentle as possible on affected areas.

Hand care

Use sunscreen and apply lotion after washing your hands (yes, every time) and at night to prevent dryness. Try a cuticle oil to keep your nails and cuticles healthy. It doesn't matter what oil you use (within reason), the main thing is to keep nails and cuticles moisturised. Don't take biotin unless you're deficient and have discussed this with your doctor (see Chapter 16).

—

When applying your body skincare, look out for any changes and see your doctor if something doesn't feel right. Yep, I'm talking about skin cancer self-checking. Use the SkinVision app to document any skin changes.

Hair removal

If you choose to remove body hair, here are some handy tips.

Shaving

Many of us shave to remove hair. It's important to wash the skin first and replace your razor blades regularly (i.e. every three uses if you don't shave daily or weekly if you do). Otherwise bacteria and dead skin will build up, which can irritate your skin or cause infection. Tap water will rinse the blade but it won't disinfect it – tap water is not sterile. Try soaking your razor blade in rubbing alcohol (60–75%) for a few minutes after use (I learned this tip from @seangarrette) and store it in a dry area. Bacteria love damp environments.

Any cleanser or shaving gel will help the razor blade glide, but be careful with thick oils and blends, particularly if they contain castor oil or coconut oil – those can clog pores. I learned this the hard way. Remember, shaving exfoliates your skin so you don't need to exfoliate again that day. It might sting if you do.

Finally, finish with some lightweight hydration – I recommend an essence or gel – and always use SPF if you'll be exposed to sun.

Shaving does not mean hair will grow back thicker. It makes the tip of the hair blunt where you cut it so it appears or feels coarser, but it won't affect the thickness of the hair. That would mean all you'd have to do to grow back a bald patch would be to shave it. See? Silly.

Epilation

An epilator is a device that looks like an electric razor, only instead of blades there are rows of tiny tweezers, to pull the hair out as it glides along. The secret to using one in the least painful way possible is to do it in the bath or shower, after the skin and hair have soaked and softened up a bit. But watch out for your ankles at the front – ouch! Epilation reduces hair growth over time, like waxing and plucking your eyebrows.

Waxing

Waxing at home can be messy but all it takes is practice. For longer lasting results, grow your hair for 4–6 weeks before waxing. My best tip is to keep the area well exfoliated right up to the day before your wax so the wax sticks to hair and not dead skin. Skip exfoliation the day of the wax, then exfoliate gently the day after. This will help prevent ingrown hairs.

Remove the wax against the hair growth (at a 180-degree angle) so as not to break the hairs. The reason why waxing reduces hair growth over time is because of the continued trauma to the hair follicle.

Laser

Laser can be thought of as permanent hair reduction.
It essentially produces hair loss for a few months and works
by selectively targeting the colour molecules in the hairs and
destroying the hair-producing stem cells in the hair follicle. You
have to catch the hair at the right part of the growth cycle, which
is why you need a few treatments per area. Your practitioner
should tell you what precautions to take leading up to your first
appointment. It does hurt a bit, especially if you've scheduled
the treatment during or close to your period. Skin can be irritated
post-laser and is best treated with a lightweight, soothing lotion.

Ingrown hairs

The key to preventing ingrowns is regular exfoliation. No picking,
or you'll be at risk of scars. You can remove ingrowns with clean,
sharp tweezers (you're allowed only two attempts). Exfoliate
every day or second day with a chemical exfoliant lotion or body
wash, and use a once-weekly treatment.

Hyperpigmentation

Hyperpigmentation on the body is much like on the face. The
causes are inflammation (this can also be friction; for example,
in the underarm area) and sun damage, and you must reduce sun
exposure to prevent progression. Incorporate a sunscreen, gentle
body exfoliants (so skin doesn't become inflamed) and active
body creams. Alternatively, use inexpensive face products on
your body.

Note that it's completely normal to have darker underarms
or other parts of the body due to the friction experienced in
these areas.

Keratosis pilaris

This is when your skin makes too much keratin and forms visibly hardened plugs. It is usually seen in the hair follicles on the backs of arms but it can also appear on the face. Use a chemically exfoliating body wash to treat the area. Because the skin on your body is thicker, it can require more exfoliation so daily use is fine. You can also use an exfoliating lotion if a wash isn't enough. Look for lactic acid, salicylic acid and urea ingredients.

Eczema

Eczema is genetic, so learning to manage it will help. Chat to your doctor or pharmacist, especially before using steroid creams. Eczema occurs because the skin isn't good at maintaining its barrier. Once the barrier is compromised, things can get in deeper and start to irritate the skin. This sets off an inflammatory cascade, resulting in an itchy, painful rash.

Here are some body care tips to keep your barrier in the best shape possible:

— **Shower or bathe in lukewarm water.** Overly hot water is drying for all skin types. Try adding a colloidal oatmeal wash to the bath.
— **Moisturise daily and immediately after bathing while skin is still damp to seal in water for maximum moisture.** Look for cleansing and moisturising products that contain ceramides, cholesterol and free fatty acids, as well as occlusives such as mineral oil. Occlusives create a fake barrier to act in place of a damaged one and can prevent a stinging sensation.
— **Don't exfoliate the eczema-prone areas.** Hydrate instead. This will help normalise your skin's shedding.

MY FAVOURITE ECZEMA PRODUCTS

Occlusive balms
— QV With Ceramides Sting-Free Ointment
— CeraVe Healing Ointment
— Vaseline Petroleum Jelly

Healing ointments
— La Roche-Posay Cicaplast Baume B5
— Avène Cicalfate Restorative Skin Cream

Moisturisers
— Bioderma Atoderm Intensive Balm
— Avène Cicalfate Restorative Skin Cream
— QV Intensive Lotion with Ceramides

Washes
— Bioderma Atoderm Shower Oil
— La Roche-Posay Lipikar Shower Oil
— QV Intensive with Ceramides Body Cleanser
— CeraVe Hydrating Cleanser
— Avène XeraCalm AD Cleansing Oil

Avoid shower oils in your later years. They can be slippery and you might be at risk of a fall.

Body breakouts

Body breakouts occur due to the same reasons as facial breakouts — trapped sweat and oil, clogged pores, inflammation and your own particular oil chemistry (influenced by genetics and hormones).

Treatment options are similar but because the body can be tedious to treat, it's important to find something simple that you'll stick to. My go-to is an exfoliating wash, especially after a workout. (Always try to shower immediately after working out.) There are also body sprays available with acids in them, and lotions with acids or retinoids. Avoid using a scrub on body acne as scrubbing will exacerbate the inflammation.

If body acne is affecting your self-esteem or you're at risk of scarring, see a doctor or dermatologist. Don't downplay it.

MY FAVOURITE BODY EXFOLIANTS

I wouldn't bother with a physical exfoliant for the body unless it contains acids as well, but I've listed some scrubs if you enjoy the sensation. The skin is just too thick and a chemical/physical mix will give a more even result.

Washes

— CeraVe SA Smoothing Cleanser
— Mecca Athletica Skin Perfecting Body Wash (AU)

Treatments and scrubs

— DDG Alpha Beta Exfoliating Body Treatment
— Alpha-H Glycolic Scrub
— Skinstitut Glycolic Scrub
— First Aid Beauty Bump Eraser KP Scrub

Lotions

— Frank Body Smoothing AHA Body Lotion
— REN AHA Smart Renewal Body Serum
— Mecca Athletica Ultra-Firming Body Lotion
— CeraVe SA Smoothing Cream

Foot care

The skin on your feet is meant to be thicker so don't file it all off. Leave those callus razors for the professionals.

MY FAVOURITE FOOT CREAMS

— Soap and Glory Heel Genius Foot Cream: Uses urea to encourage exfoliation and will sort out dry, cracked heels within a couple of days
— CeraVe SA Renewing Foot Cream: Fragrance-free and supports your barrier with ceramides as it exfoliates with salicylic acid

Deodorant

When you sweat, bacteria on your skin eat the sweat and their waste products give off a scent. Eccrine sweat is secreted all over your body, while apocrine sweat occurs after puberty in areas with more hair, such as the underarms and groin.

Some deodorants just mask the scent (essentially covering the sweat with perfume) and can be easily overwhelmed. Antiperspirants with aluminium, however, block the sweat gland to prevent the bacteria from having their food in the first place. Unless you are allergic to aluminium, these antiperspirants are fine to use; there's no medical issue with blocking the sweat gland and clinical-strength formulas are available at pharmacies. Some people also get Botox in their underarms to treat excess sweating.

MY FAVOURITE DEODORANTS

- Rexona Clinical Protection Antiperspirant Cream: Very effective and you can even apply it the night before, to avoid getting it on your clothes
- Kosas AHA deodorant: Try this if you are allergic to aluminium; it works because of the AHAs, which influence your skin's pH in a way that prevents bacteria from growing and giving off a scent

Cellulite

Most women and some men have cellulite. It's normal. People who matter do not notice you have it, or they don't care.

Cellulite appears when fat cells have poked through the hypodermis and into the dermis. There are fibrous bands of collagen called septae and these connect skin from the dermis to the muscle fascia underneath. The bands become too fibrous and tighten in an irregular way, so you end up with pockets of visibly shortened connective bands (dimples). It's not related to the thickness of the layer of fat and it's not related to your weight; in fact, liposuction can make it visibly worse because it can leave scar tissue, which is fibrous collagen too.

It seems the reason that this happens mostly to women is because the bands are perpendicular to the skin's surface, whereas for men they're more on a 45-degree angle. Rude.

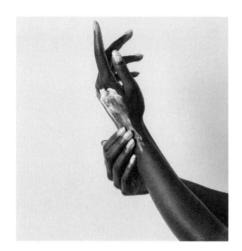
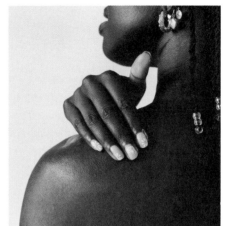
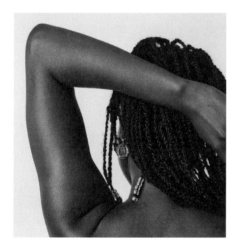
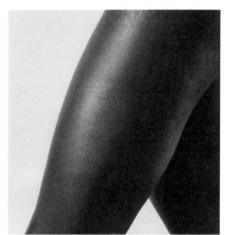

So why are we so obsessed with getting rid of cellulite?

I want you to think about where this messaging comes from and who it benefits. For years, the media, beauty industry and patriarchy have relentlessly told us that we're not good enough. We buy into that messaging and start projecting it on to ourselves and on to others. We're doing the job for them, and they start us at a young age so we don't have the tools to question or fight it.

Think about this: if a cream that got rid of cellulite existed, *no one* would have cellulite.

Key takeaways

— Your body has skin that also requires love and care.

— Put unwanted facial products to good use on your body. The skin on your body is 2–3 times thicker than the face and turns over more slowly so you can afford to be more aggressive with it (unless it's eczema-prone).

— Keep an eye out for changes on your body and see your doctor if something doesn't feel right.

— Repeat after me: cellulite is completely normal.

Injectables

[CHAPTER 18]

Before we dive into injectables, I want to have a quick word on 'ageing gracefully'. You do not have to age gracefully. You do not have to age in a way that others perceive as acceptable. Your face and body are going to change. It will happen to all of us. You are allowed to get older. The societal and media obsession with 'ageing' is judgemental and gratuitous. It's an unfair pressure, placed disproportionately on women, and I deeply resent it.

I, for one, plan to age as DISgracefully as possible.

It's no one else's business what treatments you choose to have, if any at all. You don't have to tell anyone if you don't want to, but similarly it's nothing to be ashamed of.

Having injectables is a choice. You can choose to get it, not get it, or you can get it then stop. It's a medical procedure with risks. But if you're curious, read on.

What can injectables do that skincare can't?

As you know, exposure to the sun is responsible for most of the age-related changes to your skin. Skincare and skincare ingredients can and do change the way your skin behaves. For example, retinoids can help organise the structural proteins and signal skin to hydrate itself. This means skin will look more plump and bouncy. Retinoids can also signal cells to turn over more quickly. Again, this leads to smoother-looking skin and minimised pore appearance over time. A reduction in redness and hyperpigmentation can be achieved with skincare and in-clinic treatments such as laser, peels or IPL.

But there's also fat, muscle and bone under your skin and these affect your appearance when they change and move around. For example, as you age the muscle above the top lip gets bigger and stronger and it curls the lip in and under. The forehead muscle and the muscle between the brows also get bigger and stronger, making the brows and outer corners of the eyes sit lower. Finally, the jaw becomes less angular and more square as the jaw muscles grow from years of chewing (and clenching and grinding). Your face loses supporting fat all over, with remaining fat sitting lower. You also lose some bone at the eye socket, cheek and jaw.

These changes can't be targeted with skincare. They're not skin! That's where injectables come in.

Neuromodulators

You may have heard of the brand names Botox, Dysport, Xeomin or Jeuveau – but they're all essentially the same thing: botulinum toxin. Botulinum toxina is a neurotoxic protein that comes from the bacteria clostridium botulinum and it works by blocking the signal between the nerve and muscle. This prevents the muscle from contracting and effectively paralyses the muscle depending on the dose. The injection wears off in 2–6 months, depending on the amount administered and the size and strength of the target muscle, among other things. The toxin becomes inactive and your body regenerates the nerve, then it's business as usual for that muscle. Of course, it will have become weaker in the meantime as it hasn't been used for a while, but this can be a good thing – the line might not come back for a while after the toxin wears off. When a muscle isn't used and weakens, it also shrinks, and this can change the shape of your face.

Temporarily paralysing a muscle can be a useful medical treatment for a whole host of issues. Neurologists use it to treat migraine, muscle twitches, palsies, and you can even get it for excessive sweating in underarms or feet. I swear by it for my tension headaches – can't create tense muscles if you can't tense that muscle!

The muscles around the lips also get stronger and pull lips inward as we age. Placing neuromodulators in this area ('lip flip') pushes them out again, making them look fuller.

How does this prevent or erase wrinkles?

As far as lines go, it means you can't repeatedly make the same line-forming expression. A wrinkle forms as a result of the expressions you make and loss of elasticity in the skin. By freezing the muscle, you treat the expression, and by using skincare you can treat the elasticity, to an extent.

Let's use the forehead as an example. When you raise your eyebrows as part of your normal expressions, the skin moves with it and folds. Over time (and sun exposure), the skin loses elasticity and thus the ability to bounce back to its smooth state. By paralysing the muscle underneath, we can prevent or soften the crinkling and allow skin some time to bounce back.

Fillers

Fillers usually treat lost volume in the face (or even hands) and is often just modified hyaluronic acid. There are fat pads under our skin – in our cheeks, temples and under our eyes – that move and shrink as we age. Well-placed fillers give support to the skin which might otherwise look sunken or slack. They're also used to smooth acne scars and wrinkles.

Hyaluronic acid fillers are a clear gel (like the hyaluronic acid that already exists in our bodies), only they're modified to take longer to break down so that the effect of the filler lasts six months to two years (but they can stay in your body for longer than that). Hyaluronic acid fillers also vary in thickness, so you might want a thicker one for the cheek, but something thinner for the lips.

Lips thin in appearance as we age due to loss of structural proteins (collagen) and loss of hydration (reduction of hyaluronic acid). A filler can revolumise and rehydrate lips, which isn't something you can do as dramatically with skincare.

If you're after something subtler and longer lasting, there are other kinds of fillers that work in different ways such as collagen-stimulating fillers (poly-l-lactic acid/Sculptra) and calcium hydroxyapatite (Radiesse).

Fat-dissolving injections

Also known under the brand name Kybella/Belkyra, fat-dissolving injections are made from a copy of your bile salts (deoxycholic acid), which help to dissolve the fats that you digest. It is injected into the fat under your chin (and apparently feels like burning), causes swelling and destroys some of the fat cells, thus reducing the look of a 'double chin'. You normally need a few treatments for a good result and it's quite expensive per visit.

Hyaluronic acid is very good at grabbing and holding on to water, so staying hydrated can actually give your fillers a more volumised look.

Regulations and choosing the right practitioner

In Australia, anti-wrinkle injections and filler must be prescribed and administered by a registered medical professional. Doctors and dentists can prescribe, while nurses can administer under doctor supervision. You can check their registration via the AHPRA database. Injectables are classed as prescription-only medicines, such as an antidepressant or the contraceptive pill. It's important for injectables to be administered by medical professionals as they're not only experienced in administering them, but also in what to do if something goes wrong. In the US it's much the same but it can vary between states. In the UK, however, there's minimal regulation for non-surgical cosmetic interventions. While doctors must prescribe them, anyone can legally administer Botox and fillers.

In terms of safety, it's not only about practical training but also the medical knowledge and knowledge of facial anatomy that underpins it. If you choose to have injectable cosmetic interventions, please make sure you get your treatments from a safe provider. If the price seems too good to be true, it probably is.

I haven't found much of a difference in my own post-treatment satisfaction between doctors, nurses and dentists for injectables, but my advice is to choose someone who is experienced and whose work you like. Make sure they understand the results you're after and that they're realistic. These settings can leave us vulnerable so you want someone who is kind and who you can trust. The last thing I want is a practitioner pointing out things I hadn't noticed or using unkind language.

If you have a friend or follow someone on social media and you like the work they've had done, ask them (politely!) who they see and what they thought. Some practitioners have a great eye for it. Ask how they feel about their treatment after it's settled in for a little while, not on the day of the procedure. Filler can move where it's not meant to. However, with correct placement and an experienced, well-trained practitioner, the risk is minimal.

If you choose to have injectable cosmetic interventions, please make sure you get your treatments from a safe provider. If the price seems too good to be true, it probably is.

Key takeaways

— Injectables are medical procedures and no one is obligated to disclose if they've had work done.

— Don't shame people for getting treatments. We can't speculate on how much someone's mental health, or even employment, is affected by beauty standards.

— Conversely, don't shame people for not getting treatments either.

— Do not be seduced by cheap 'deals' – spend time researching. This is your face.

The comparison trap and self-care

[CHAPTER 19]

I take and post pictures of my face a lot (occupational hazard) and sometimes I still get upset looking at my own face from a year ago. Even though I know it's my best angle in the shot, that it took me at least two hours of hair and makeup, not to mention maybe an hour the previous day to exfoliate and apply self-tanner. Then there's the hour earlier in the week I spent perming and tinting my eyebrows. And the manicure I got the previous weekend. That's without starting on skincare, facials, in-clinic skin treatments … and photo editing.

Think about it this way: if I asked you to draw yourself and you're not well practised at drawing, what you produce might not be very accurate. But you wouldn't look at the sketch and say, 'I look bad', right? You'd say, 'I can't draw.' It's the same for photos. People who are photographed often, such as models, have practised – a lot. And more often than not it's about the skill of the photographer and not about *you*.

These photos are from the same day. See how the harsh overhead lighting creates shadows, whereas the soft, diffused light makes things more even and smooth? If you know what you're doing, you can manipulate things accordingly to achieve the effect you want.

It's not unusual for advertisements to have had hours of retouching work done, to brighten eyes and teeth and improve skin texture, to make skin look perfect without looking fake (sometimes ...).

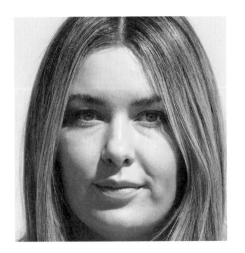
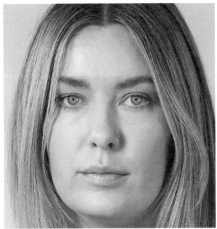

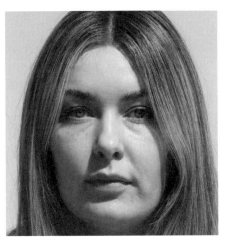
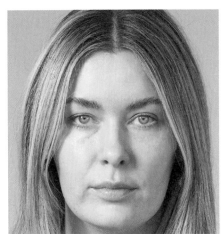

Sure, it's compelling to view an ad with a before and after photo, but the lighting could be different, the skin could be more moisturised, the angle more flattering ... and you also don't know what else has changed for that person in between photos. There are many things to take into account. When skin progress is documented in a medical setting, the same camera is used in the same room with the same lighting. Sometimes a VISIA device is used, which is a machine that can photograph the pigment changes in the deeper layers of skin or where the most blood vessels are or even where there's residue from acne bacteria. You rarely see these photos in before and after Instagram ads.

Then there's the fact that many celebrities and influencers have dermatologists and facialists on call, regular in-clinic skin treatments and professional makeup application for events and photoshoots. Some have had liposuction and fat transfer, rhinoplasty (nose jobs) – everything you can imagine. You can't compare yourself to $50k of plastic surgery.

So if everyone's lying about their appearance and skin results, and crediting their radiant, ageless appearance to olive oil (never Botox), how can we cut through that noise and accept ourselves as we are?

Self-care

Self-care is a conscious effort to look after your health. This includes your emotional, mental and physical health. Sure, it can mean a soak in the bathtub with your favourite bubble bath and luxury face mask, but more often than not it's a lot less glamorous than that. It's remembering to eat and take your medicine. It's scheduling and attending doctor's appointments. It's seeing friends. It's getting your steps in, if you're able to. Self-care is an ongoing commitment.

Self-care checklist

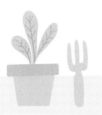
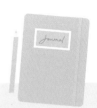

- GARDENING

- WATCH A FAVOURITE MOVIE

- EAT A NUTRITIOUS SNACK

- DRINK WATER

- BATH OR SHOWER

- READ A BOOK

- MOVE MY BODY

- DO MY MAKEUP FOR FUN

- WRITE IN MY JOURNAL

- PLAN SOMETHING FUN
  (HOLIDAY, ART GALLERY VISIT)

- TAKE A NAP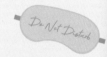

- GET OUT OF THE HOUSE

- COLLAGE FROM MAGAZINES

- BEYONCÉ DANCE PARTY

- DIGITAL DETOX

Be mindful of what you take on

Does this scenario sound familiar? You've just woken up, reach for your phone and start scrolling through social media. You're not really paying attention, just going through the motions. Half-an-hour passes and you start feeling upset. Did you wake up feeling this way? Or did you take on something while scrolling?

For me, it's usually something I took on and it takes a while to track down the source. The solution is to think about the accounts you're following. Social media can be harmful to your mind and it's super helpful to curate your experience while on these platforms. Interact with the accounts you enjoy, that make you feel good – comment, like, save, reply to stories, share with your friends. Mute or unfollow the ones that don't make you feel good. You don't owe anyone your time or views.

I can't take on content that perpetuates diet culture. Before and after weight loss? No. Calorie counting? Don't think so. I highly recommend pressing 'not interested' on TikTok and Instagram if things you don't want to see come up on your pages. What do you love seeing on your social media feeds? Search for it and let it nourish your mind.

Happy list

Sometimes negative feelings are hard to shake. If it's been two weeks or more then it might be helpful to speak to a professional – ask a trusted family member or friend to help you find one if needed. You're allowed to feel sad and to take your time to process those feelings, but when you don't want to feel sad anymore, ask yourself what makes you happy? What clears your head? Write it all down in a happy list and refer to it when you need a reset.

Here's my happy list. You don't have to do everything! They're just suggestions of things I find calming or inspiring that feed my mind. I'll do one or two of these things if I'm feeling low.

— Gardening
— Watching my favourite movie

— Eating a nutritious snack
— Drinking water
— Bathing or showering
— Reading a book
— Moving my body
— Jigsaw puzzle
— Doing my makeup for fun
— Writing in my journal
— Planning something (holiday, art gallery visit)
— Taking a nap
— Getting out of the house
— Crafting
— Collaging from magazines
— Beyoncé dance party
— Digital detox

At the end of the day, your skin is the interface between you and the outside world – it's how people see you, it's how you see yourself, and it makes sense to start your care regimen and relationship with yourself right here. It's not about how you look, it's about acceptance and being comfortable within your own skin.

I hope that by understanding your skin, you can understand and be kinder to yourself.

THE COMPARISON TRAP AND SELF-CARE

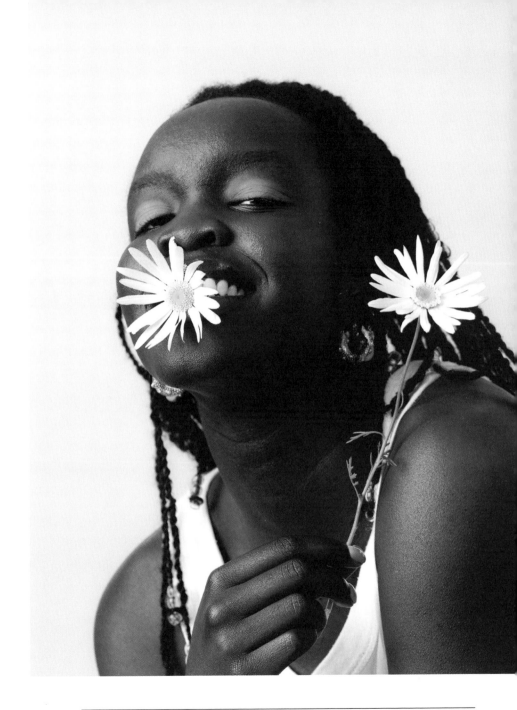

Glossary

Actives

In pharmaceuticals, the 'active' ingredient(s) in a product are the ones doing the medicating, while the others are called 'excipients'. For example, in an exfoliating serum, the actives are the ingredients that exfoliate; in a moisturiser, the actives add moisture.

In skincare, actives can also refer to ingredients that are a bit 'spicy' for your skin, ones that must be approached carefully. For example, if you have a microneedling treatment and they tell you 'no actives for a week', this would mean no vitamin A and derivatives, exfoliating products of any kind (acid, enzyme, scrub), vitamin C (specifically L-ascorbic acid), hydroquinone or prescription skincare creams, unless otherwise directed.

AHAs

Alpha hydroxy acids are exfoliating acids that can increase sun sensitivity, so be sure to slip, slop, slap for a week after using them.

Antioxidant

Antioxidants are molecules that are great at reacting with free radicals (unstable molecules) so your DNA and cell membranes don't have to, ensuring that free radicals can't destabilise and derail your skin's function. They offer protection so you can use your energy to heal on a molecular level. The more antioxidants you have in your life, the better. Lots of ingredients have antioxidant properties and it generally means they are soothing to the skin – they're extra brilliant paired with sunscreen.

BHAs

Beta hydroxy acids are oil-soluble exfoliating acids, which are great for use in oily areas. Unlike AHAs, they do not increase sun sensitivity.

Emulsifier

An emulsifier is a type of surfactant that helps mix things together that wouldn't otherwise mix. Its job in personal care products is to stabilise the oil and water phases so the product doesn't separate.

Enzyme

An enzyme is a protein, but not all proteins are enzymes. Specifically, enzymes are proteins that facilitate a reaction. They're involved in thousands of biological reactions and the molecule that the enzyme acts on is called a substrate. Exfoliating enzymes break down proteins such as the keratin in the top layers of corneocytes.

Essence

An essence falls somewhere between a serum and a toner in terms of ingredient concentration and thickness (or viscosity). It usually contains fermented ingredients.

Eye cream

An eye cream is a moisturiser that has been tested for eye safety. The eye area has unique concerns as the skin is thinner there.

Face oil

A facial oil is a great way to amp up your moisturiser in the winter or get a very glowy look. The idea is to add a safe, non-clogging oil to your face, to help repel water back into your skin, thus slowing the loss of moisture throughout the day. Certain oils have properties that can also help to balance your natural oils. You might see the words 'hydrating face oil', but the key to good hydration is a good blend of humectants and emollients or occlusives. Face oils are usually just concentrated emollients. Some oils might say 'brightening' or 'acne preventing' but if you're struggling with acne or hyperpigmentation, a face oil won't cut it (unless it contains proven ingredients for those concerns).

Facial device

Fancy devices are fun. They're also usually pricey. My advice: no dermabrasion and strictly no harsh, scrubby brushes with bristles. Get a set of super-soft washcloths instead. Microcurrent and ultrasound devices are great (so is LED), but if you're not going to use them regularly (i.e. 3–5 times a week), they're not worth it and you won't see results.

Ferment

When something ferments, it changes due to yeast or bacteria. In skincare, ingredients are fermented to extract different things. Fermented ingredients help to reduce sensitivity, gently brighten skin and support the microbiome.

Free radicals

Free radicals are unstable molecules. They're a normal part of our body's metabolism but they can react with important structures in our cells and skin, damaging and destabilising them. There are free radicals in air pollution and they're also generated by UV radiation hitting our skin. Free radicals can be neutralised by antioxidants, which is why we're so obsessed with antioxidants in skincare.

Glycation

Glycation occurs when free sugars (e.g. glucose or fructose) attach to proteins (e.g. collagen and elastin) or lipids. This process can't be reversed and over time the collagen becomes less flexible. It's not about what you eat – sugars are part of our metabolism and their accumulation in proteins is a fact of life. Using skincare with antioxidants or ingredients with anti-glycation properties can help slow this process down.

Lipids

Lipids are a class of organic (biological) molecules that includes fatty acids (e.g. omega-3s), sterols (e.g. cholesterol), waxes (e.g. ceramides), triglycerides, fat-soluble vitamins (e.g. vitamin A) and phospholipids. A key characteristic of lipids is that they won't easily dissolve in water. Imagine oil floating on top of water. Our cell membranes are made of lipids.

Mask

A mask is a skincare treatment designed for use 1–2 times a week. Sheet masks are essentially a large amount of serum that you press in to your face with the piece of cotton, allowing it to absorb more deeply. They are usually hydrating. Clay masks are designed to draw excess debris from your pores. Moisturising and calming masks are moisturisers that you wash off. Sleeping masks are moisturisers designed to be applied before bed and usually create a seal to prevent everything else on your skin from evaporating. Exfoliating and peeling masks can be quite strong.

Moisturiser

A moisturiser is a cream with both water and oil-based ingredients, designed to help support your skin's barrier and prevent water loss.

NMF

Your skin's natural moisturising factors. These are water-grabbing molecules that help to hydrate.

Occlusive

An occlusive ingredient is a thick ingredient, often found in balms or ointments, that forms a physical barrier to act in place of the natural barrier. Occlusion means 'blockage' in medicine.

Peptide

Broadly speaking, a peptide is a chain of 2–50 amino acids. In skincare, a peptide can do several things: some are antioxidants (e.g. glutathione), some signal skin to repair (e.g. matrixyl) and some are antibacterial (oligopeptide-76). There are also neuropeptides such as argireline – or 'Botox in a bottle' – that work to prevent muscle contraction, thus reducing wrinkles. Peptides such as soybean peptides inhibit enzymes, which prevent collagen from being unnecessarily broken down. Some peptides are better researched than others and you only need a very small amount in your skincare product (parts-per-million small).

Protein

A protein is a 3D structure made up of 50 or more amino acids. Proteins do lots of things. Collagen is a protein, our muscles are made of proteins (called actin and myosin) and insulin is a protein too. What's important to know about proteins in relation to skincare is that they're too big to be absorbed into skin and the ones already in our skin are not fans of the sun, free radicals or glycation.

Serum

A serum is a concentrated, usually water-based way to deliver targeted ingredients to your skin. Serums can do all kinds of things – exfoliate, brighten, improve texture, reduce redness, protect from the environment and hydrate. If you have a defined skincare goal in mind, a serum can be incorporated to help you achieve that goal.

Spot treatment

Spot treatments work by delivering ingredients directly to the blemish. You can spot treat many things – breakouts, dryness and even dark spots.

Toner

Toner can refer to many things but the constant is that it's a very liquid, almost watery texture. Toners used to be harsh and often stripping (some still are), but these days you can find toners that hydrate, mattify or exfoliate. Toner is a good way to deliver ingredients to your skin without feeling heavy. Think of it as a very watery serum and choose one for your needs.

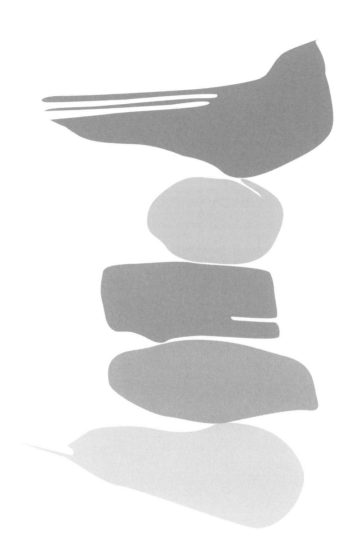

Endnotes

1 Gebauer, K. (2017). Acne in adolescents. *Australian Family Physician*, *46*(12), 892–895.

2 Brown, H., Tapley, A., van Driel, M., Davey, A., Holliday, E., Ball, J., Morgan, S., Patsan, I., Mulquiney, K., Spike, N., FitzGerald, K., & Magin, P. (2019). Acne in primary care: A cross-sectional analysis. *Australian Journal of General Practice*, *48*(11), 781–788.

3 Pazyar, N., Yaghoobi, R., Bagherani, N., & Kazerouni, A. (2012). A review of applications of tea tree oil in dermatology. *International Journal of Dermatology*, *52*(7), 784–790.

4 Koo, J. (1995). The psychosocial impact of acne: Patients' perceptions. *Journal of the American Academy of Dermatology*, *32*(5), S26–30.

5 Hinkley, S. B., Holub, S. C., & Menter, A. (2020). The validity of cutaneous body image as a construct and as a mediator of the relationship between cutaneous disease and mental health. *Dermatology and Therapy*, *10*(1), 203–211.

6 Jafferany, M. (2007). Psychodermatology. *The Primary Care Companion to the Journal of Clinical Psychiatry*, *9*(3), 203–213.

7 Giacomoni, P. U., Mammone, T., & Teri, M. (2009). Gender-linked differences in human skin. *Journal of Dermatological Science*, *55*(3), 144–149.

8 Halprin, K. M. (1972). Epidermal 'turnover time' – a re-examination. *British Journal of Dermatology*. January.

9 Cichorek, M., Wachulska, M., Stasiewicz, A., & Tymińska, A. (2013). Skin melanocytes: Biology and development. *Postepy Dermatol Alergo*l, *30*(1), 30–41.

10 Wang, X., Yuan, C., & Humbert, P. (2017). Evaluation of skin surface flora, *Agache's Measuring the Skin*, 107–112.

11 Further reading: Singh, N. (2020, August 13). Decolonising dermatology: Why black and brown skin need better treatment. *The Guardian*. www.theguardian.com/society/2020/aug/13/decolonising-dermatology-why-black-and-brown-skin-need-better-treatment

12 Oakley, A. (2012). *Fitzpatrick skin phototype.* DermNet NZ. https://dermnetnz.org/topics/skin-phototype/

13 Farage, M. A. (2019). The prevalence of sensitive skin. *Frontiers in Medicine, 6,* 98.

14 SunSmart Australia. (n.d.). *Skin cancer stats & facts.* www.sunsmart.com.au/skin-cancer/skin-cancer-facts-stats

15 Hughes, M. C. B., Williams, G. M., Baker, P., & Green, A. C. (2013). Sunscreen and prevention of skin aging: A randomized trial. *Ann Intern Med, 158*(11), 781–790.

16 Kaidbey, K. H., Agin, P. P., Sayre, R. M., & Kligman, A. M. (1979). Photoprotection by melanin – a comparison of black and Caucasian skin. *Journal of the American Academy of Dermatology, 1*(3), 249–260.

17 de Gruijl, F. R. (2000). Photocarcinogenesis: UVA vs UVB. *Methods in Enzymology, 319,* 359–366.

18 Kaidbey, K. H., Agin, P. P., Sayre, R. M., & Kligman, A. M. (1979). Photoprotection by melanin – a comparison of black and Caucasian skin. *Journal of the American Academy of Dermatology, 1*(3), 249–260.

19 Bernstein, E. F., Brown, D. B., Schwartz, M. D., Kaidbey, K., & Ksenzenko, S. M. (2004). The polyhydroxy acid gluconolactone protects against ultraviolet radiation in an in vitro model of cutaneous photoaging. *Dermatologic Surgery, 30*(2), 189–196.

20 Katiyar, S. K. (2007). UV-induced immune suppression and photocarcinogenesis: Chemoprevention by dietary botanical agents. *Cancer Letters, 255*(1), 1–11.

21 Chung, J. H., & Eun, H. C. (2007). Angiogenesis in skin aging and photoaging. *The Journal of Dermatology, 34*(9), 593–600.

22 Campiche, R., Curpen, S. J., Lutchmanen-Kolanthan, V., Gougeon, S., Cherel, M., Laurent, G., Gempeler, M., & Schuetz, R. (2020). Pigmentation effects of blue light irradiation on skin and how to protect against them. *International Journal of Cosmetic Science, 42*(4), 399–406.

23 Ou-Yang, H., Jiang, L. I., & Meyer, K. (2017). Sun protection by beach umbrella vs sunscreen with a high sun protection factor: A randomized clinical trial. *AMA Dermatol, 153*(3), 304–308.

24 Australian Government. (n.d.). *Sun protection using sunglasses.* ARPANSA. www.arpansa.gov.au/understanding-radiation/radiation-sources/more-radiation-sources/sun-protection-sunglasses

25 Holick, M. F., MacLaughlin, J. A., Clark, M. B., Holick, S. A., Potts Jr, J. T., Anderson, R. R., Blank, I. H., Parrish, J. A., & Elias, P. (1980). Photosynthesis of previtamin D3 in human skin and the physiologic consequences. *Science, 210*(4466), 203–205.

26 Norval, M., & Wulf, H. C. (2009). Does chronic sunscreen use reduce vitamin D production to insufficient levels? *British Journal of Dermatology, 161*(4), 732–736.

27 Cancer Council Australia. (2016). *Position statement: Sun exposure and vitamin D – risks and benefits.* https://wiki.cancer.org.au/policy/Position_ statement_-_Risks_and_benefits_of_sun_exposure#Key_messages_ and_recommendations

28 Randhawa, M., Wang, S., Leyden, J. L., Cula, G. O., Pagnoni, A., & Southall, M. D. (2016). Daily use of a facial broad spectrum sunscreen over one-year significantly improves clinical evaluation of photoaging. *Dermatol Surg, 42*(12), 1354–1361.

29 Leach, G. (2019, May 31). Meet the Kakadu plum: An international superfood thousands of years in the making. *The Conversation.* https:// theconversation.com/meet-the-kakadu-plum-an-international- superfood-thousands-of-years-in-the-making-116362

30 Alanazi, M. S., Hammad, S. M., & Mohamed, A. E. (2018). Prevalence and psychological impact of acne vulgaris among female secondary school students in Arar city, Saudi Arabia, in 2018. *Electron Physician, 10*(8), 7224–7229; Skin Health Institute. (n.d.). *Acne.* www.skinhealthinstitute. org.au/page/89/acne

31 Clearihan, L. (2001). Acne: Myths and management issues. *Australian Family Physician, 30*(11), 1039–1044.

32 Felmingham, C., Kerr, A., & Veysey, E. (2020). Costs incurred by patients with acne prior to dermatological consultation and their relation to patient income. *Australasian Journal of Dermatology, 61*(4), 384–386.

33 NSW Government. (2021). Skin care, hair care and cosmetic treatments in pregnancy and breastfeeding. MotherSafe – Royal Hospital for Women. www.seslhd.health.nsw.gov.au/sites/default/files/groups/Royal_ Hospital_for_Women/Mothersafe/documents/skinhairpregbr2021.pdf

34 Baldwin, H., & Tan, J. (2021). Effects of diet on acne and its response to treatment. *American Journal of Clinical Dermatology, 22*(1), 55–65.

35 Choi, F. D., Sung, C. T., Juhasz, M. L., & Mesinkovsk, N. A. (2019). Oral collagen supplementation: A systematic review of dermatological applications. *Journal of Drugs in Dermatology, 18*(1), 9–16.

Thank you

To the scientists, clinicians and doctors that tirelessly fact-check and educate, for free, on social media.

To Michelle Wong, specifically – your work has changed so much of our industry and held it accountable, thank you. You never miss.

To Alice Hardie-Grant and Camha Pham, thank you for making my work the best it can be, and for your vision.

To Ava Matthews, Bec Jefferd, Melissa Hennessy, thank you for everything, really. I am honoured to know you and cannot overstate how much it means to me.

To Noelle Faulkner. I couldn't have done it without you. You are the coolest, endlessly empathetic, and my cherished friend.

To Alice Kenyon, my fabulous manager and cheerleader, the real brains of the operation.

To Clary, Bianca, Liz, for hearing me out and for being happy for me – it means so much.

To Mum, Dad, Clare, Max, for knowing me better than I know myself and reminding me that I can do this, and that it's pretty great.

To my wonderful partner, Ryan. Thank you for believing in me before I did. Thank you for your encouragement, patience, kindness, for being there for me through all the late nights and weekends, for tirelessly making sure I ate and slept well throughout the process. For faithfully wearing your sunscreen without me having to ask. This is your work just as much as it's mine. I love you, thank you.

About the author

Hannah English is a beauty writer and content creator with a background in pharmaceutical research. An enthusiastic communicator, she has built a niche within the beauty industry around her passion for making science feel cool, relevant and accessible. Like many teens, Hannah grew up with acne and low self-esteem, with few scientific solutions made available to her. This is what led her to study pharmaceutical science, and today, she shares everything she knows to make sure her experience as a young person is one of the past. Armed with this knowledge and her razor-sharp view on the wider beauty and skincare landscape, Hannah is peeling back the label to reveal the truth, and to educate and help everyone to best understand and protect the skin they're in.

Index

Published in 2022 by Hardie Grant Books, an imprint of Hardie Grant Publishing

Hardie Grant Books (Melbourne)
Wurundjeri Country
Building 1, 658 Church Street
Richmond, Victoria 3121

Hardie Grant Books (London)
5th & 6th Floors
52–54 Southwark Street
London SE1 1UN

hardiegrantbooks.com

 A catalogue record for this
book is available from the
National Library of Australia

Your Best Skin
ISBN 9781743797693

10 9 8 7 6 5 4 3 2 1

Commissioning Editor: Alice Hardie-Grant
Editor: Camha Pham
Design Manager: Kristin Thomas
Designer: Studio Polka
Typesetter: Patrick Cannon
Photographer: Becca Crawford
Stylist: Stephanie Stamatis
Production Manager: Todd Rechner
Production Coordinator: Jessica Harvie

Colour reproduction by Splitting Image Colour Studio
Printed in China by Leo Paper Products LTD.

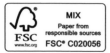 The paper this book is printed on is from FSC®-certified
forests and other sources. FSC® promotes environmentally
responsible, socially beneficial and economically viable
management of the world's forests.

Hardie Grant acknowledges the Traditional Owners of the country on which we work,
the Wurundjeri people of the Kulin nation and the Gadigal people of the Eora nation,
and recognises their continuing connection to the land, waters and culture. We pay
our respects to their Elders past and present.